T0380167

THE
BRIDAL
BLUEPRINT

HOW TO PREPARE FOR THE UNEXPECTED, DISCOVER YOUR PERSONAL STYLE AND LOOK LIKE THE BRIDE OF YOUR DREAMS

FIONA TAYLOR

© 2023 Fiona Taylor. All rights reserved.

No part of this book may be reproduced, stored in a retrieval system, or
transmitted by any means without the written permission of the author.

AuthorHouse™
1663 Liberty Drive
Bloomington, IN 47403
www.authorhouse.com
Phone: 833-262-8899

Because of the dynamic nature of the Internet, any web addresses or links contained in this book may have changed
since publication and may no longer be valid. The views expressed in this work are solely those of the author and do
not necessarily reflect the views of the publisher, and the publisher hereby disclaims any responsibility for them.

Any people depicted in stock imagery provided by Getty Images are models,
and such images are being used for illustrative purposes only.
Certain stock imagery © Getty Images.

The information in this book is for entertainment purposes only. It is not meant to diagnose any health
conditions. The information is strictly the opinion of the author. Any advice should be used with personal
discretion. The author assumes no responsibility or liability for any loss, damages or injury.

This book is printed on acid-free paper.

ISBN: 978-1-7283-7740-7 (sc)
ISBN: 978-1-7283-7742-1 (hc)
ISBN: 978-1-7283-7741-4 (e)

Library of Congress Control Number: 2023900763

Print information available on the last page.

Published by AuthorHouse 03/08/2023

authorHOUSE

THE
BRIDAL
BLUEPRINT

CONTENTS

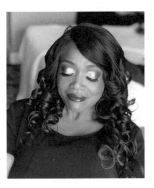 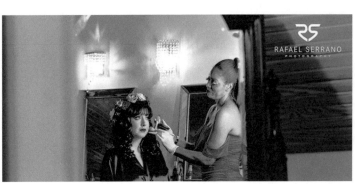 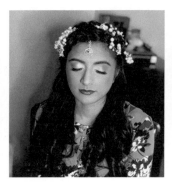

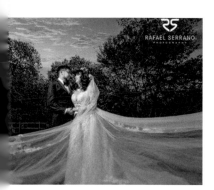
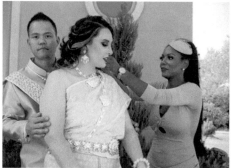
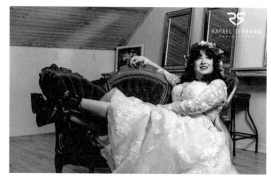

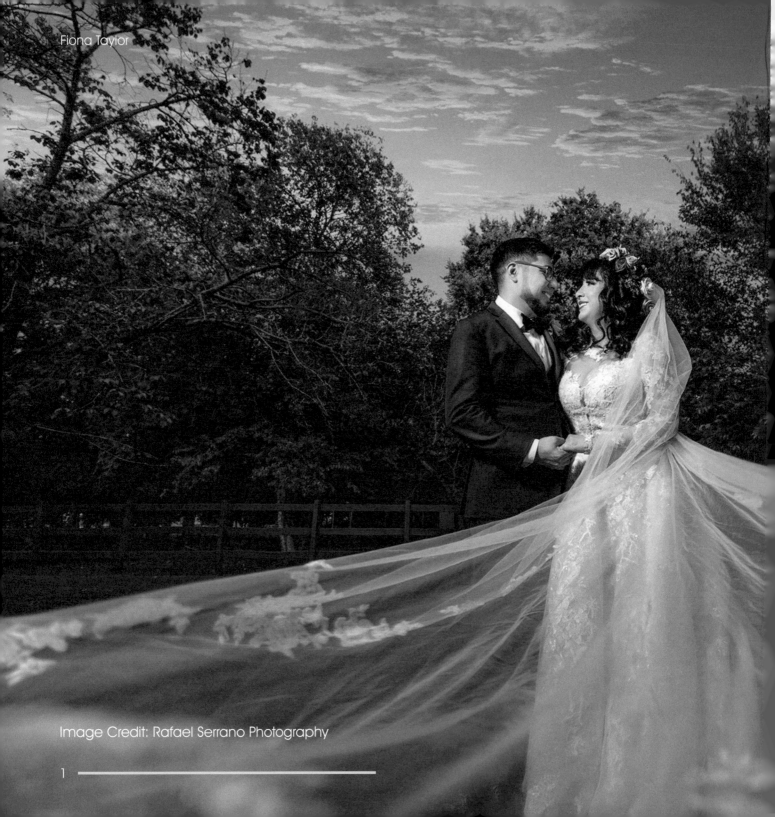

Fiona Taylor

Image Credit: Rafael Serrano Photography

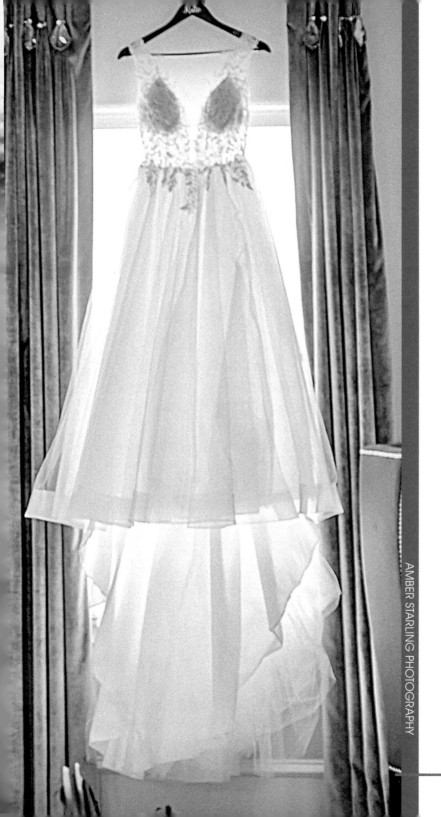

AMBER STARLING PHOTOGRAPHY

Introduction

I was mystified by the sight.

There she was… standing outside in the grueling heat of a typical Texas summer. The bride was trying to maintain her composure in 103-degree weather while wearing 20 pounds of fluff and her face—leaking like a faucet. I reacted quickly and went straight into damage control mode! This was just the beginning of her wedding day. I knew her bridal photos had to come together ASAP—so the patchwork began.

Brides find themselves panicked due to unexpected emergency situations all the time. Every bride dreams of looking absolutely amazing for their big day. It wouldn't be an overstatement to say that brides are planning to look the best they'll ever look in their life. Planning ahead for the unexpected should be one of the most important decisions for your wedding day.

The question then becomes, "How can I plan for something I've never experienced?" Even if it's your second go around, unconsidered issues can wreak havoc on your special moment and quickly spiral out of control.

This is your blueprint for navigating the most essential components of your wedding day appearance. By following the guidance in this book, you will not only look like a dreamy bride but also gain in-depth knowledge and understanding of the processes involved in achieving a perfection level found only in fairytale stories.

Having worked in careers specializing in fashion and beauty for special events permitted me to have first-hand encounters with the backstory and experiences of countless bridal clients. I've had the opportunity of working with hundreds of brides that have entrusted their appearance to my craftsmanship. My everyday experiences with clients have allowed me to analyze and dissect important elements that directly contribute to what can give the best conceivable look for their individual needs.

My passion for beauty has allowed me to successfully lead Faces by Fiona. My award-winning special event company works with luxury brides and elite clientele for various beauty needs. We deliver expert direction and prestigious beauty services for the most discerning clients who allow us to make their vision of looking elegant and feeling empowered come to life. An empowered bride exudes glamour, confidence, and sophistication. An empowered bride is a prepared bride.

Preparing to look your best is the most important journey you can take. Your appearance can boost your confidence and impact your mood and how others perceive you. #BeautyMatters

Widening your understanding of your personal tastes in beauty, proper skincare, hair maintenance, and beauty etiquette will allow you to look more polished and refined.

By reading *The Bridal Blueprint*, you will understand how to prepare for the unexpected, learn to navigate through the different aspects of your appearance, and gain insights on composure that will ensure you feel in control, confident, photograph flawlessly, and look absolutely stunning from all angles.

Learning more about what it takes to look dreamy is a process worth divining into. Waiting to begin your journey could transition into becoming an unorganized nervous wreck or, worse, finding yourself in less desirable circumstances that could've been prevented. Queue song, "It's my party."

The truth is, your friends and relatives can offer sound advice from their own priceless wedding experience. This book takes it a step further by offering years of experience, quintessential field research, and live studies compiled into a comprehensive, interactive book from an expert in the beauty industry.

Begin reading this blueprint guide to methodically prepare to show up as the most beautiful version of yourself with information that goes even further than your wedding day. This is your ticket to looking like you've stepped out of your imagination. Your journey to looking dreamy starts today!

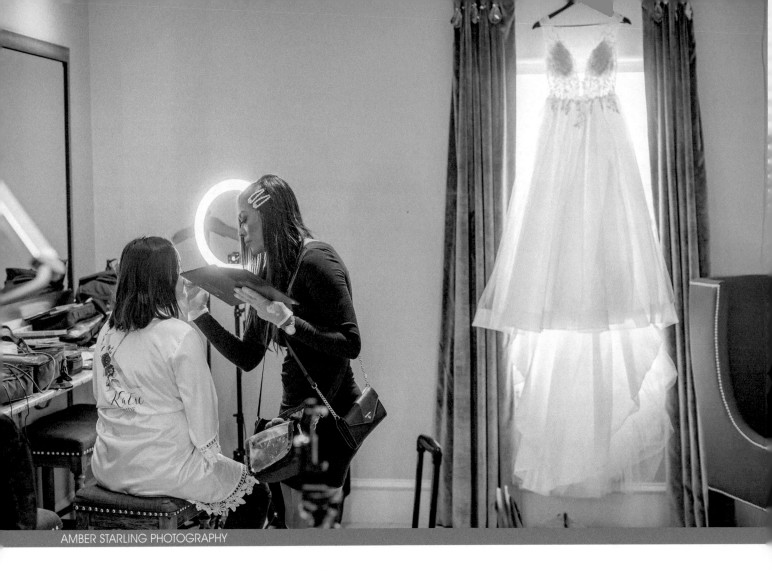

AMBER STARLING PHOTOGRAPHY

Chapter 1: About Face

We've all heard it 1000 times and then questioned what else we need to know to live up to the quote's hype…

"Great skin leads to great makeup."

Yes, the famous one-size-fits-all answer that we've heard from makeup artists at every department store counter to estheticion's in high-end spas! This statement probably left you feeling like those words are only uttered from the lips of beauty gurus with 101 different products with extreme instructions you're unlikely to consistently follow...

Fast forward to reality—You can create the skin care routine that works best for you! Let's start with the basics!! To truly have the bridal glow, you'll want to hone in on having balanced skin. In your skin care routine, you should have the following:

Basic Products

- Daily cleanser
- Toner
- Day moisturizer
- Night moisturizer
- Sunscreen
- Eye cream

Bonus Products

- Targeted treatment for main skin concerns
- Weekly exfoliator
- Weekly treatment mask
- Makeup remover

No one will know your skin like you do. The first step to finding what your skin loves and what is most beneficial to you is understanding what your skin lacks. Below, you'll find examples of how to determine what your skin is craving:

Desert Situation, Aka Dry Skin

Skin that feels tight, has flaky areas, appears dull, and is visibly scaly is thirsty and needs hydration. Products that have water-attracting qualities to nourish the skin are ideal. An ingredient like hyaluronic acid is renowned for retaining 1,000 times its weight in water.

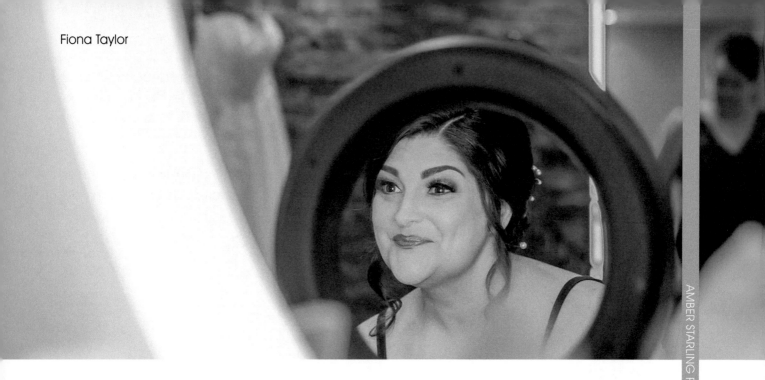

AMBER STARLING PHOTOGRAPHY

To rid the skin of rough texture or flakiness, you'll want an exfoliant that sloughs the dead skin away. It will also build the integrity of the skin by strengthening it via building elasticity with the introduction of Lactic Acid or Vitamin A. Both are amazing for relieving dry, irritated skin! With daily use, you say siñanara to lifeless skin in no time at all!

One predisposition to having a dryer skin type is its nature to crease and wrinkle. Ceramides and plant oils will keep your skin buttery smooth, literally! They work by sealing in hydrating ingredients, preventing moisture loss, and strengthening the skin's protective barrier. The less your skin is dry, the more chances you'll have to fight back from it breaking down and creasing.

Wicked Slick, Aka Oily Skin

Suppose your skin has its own natural glow that turns into a reflective shield of armor within a short time. In that case, you may be looking for ways to rescue your skin from its overproduction of oil!

Working alongside photographers has given me insight into what picks up well in photos. Most industry professionals can agree with me that having a clean and matte face overall works

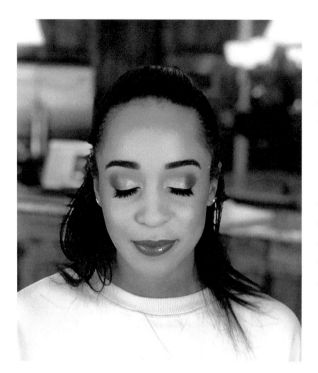

great for capturing your best bridal appearance. In addition, it's less editing work for them!

To rid skin of over production of oil, you want to start with ingredients that absorb and excavate the grime that attaches to oil that is responsible for breakouts.

Let's start with absorption. Although producing sebum is great for protecting and conditioning the skin, it can become bothersome if uncontrolled. If you can commit to a weekly skin pampering session, you'll see a diminished oily appearance. Using a clay mask works like a magnet to draw out impurities and clarify congested pores.

The acid crew: salicylic acid, glycolic acid, and lactic acid are the trio that has your back! If you've never thought rubbing acid on your face was a good idea... you're not alone! Although it may sound intimidating, incorporating one into your cleanser or opting for an after-wash toner with a clinical percentage would be ideal for keeping clean pores. Choosing a product that actively treats bacteria, sloughs dean skin away, and brightens your complexion is a perfect balance for skin with an overabundant supply of oil and/ or breaks out often.

You had me at Goodbye, aka Sensitive Skin

If you find that your skin is not very open to accepting new experiences, it may be trying to tell you it needs to stick to what

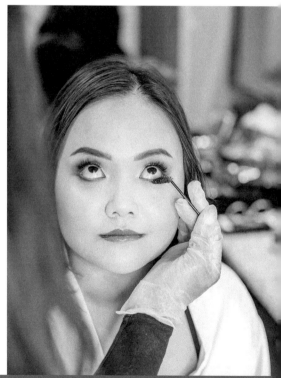

AMBER STARLING PHOTOGRAPHY

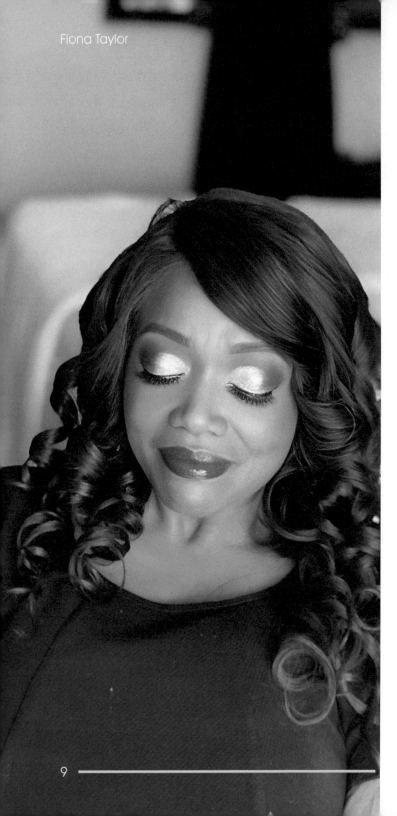

it likes! Small flare-ups with redness, burning, itchiness, and a rough texture are generally reactions you'd want to steer clear of.

Sensitive skin can be triggered by weather, genetics, the environment, and the wrong products for your skin type. Although all skin types can benefit from a skin screen, it is particularly important for your skin types as it can protect your skin and help keep it calm. Fluctuating temperatures from excessive heat to icy cold can also activate the reactions. Simply wearing protective headwear and scarves can improve your appearance if you find yourself in situations wherein changing temperatures occur.

Flakey surface texture and roughness can be a bothersome side effect of overly sensitive skin. You'll find that introducing a nourishing moisturizer that is either hypoallergenic or low in harsh fragrances can assist. A personal favorite for both an improvement of texture as well as a preventative measure is a face oil! Natural ingredients such as jojoba, vitamin E, olive-derived, and argan oils can be anti-aging and keep your skin baby smooth!

Many factors can come into play when dealing with skin issues. You'll often find that you may have concerns that overlap, which can be overwhelming. This is a normal happening. Starting with the most bothersome issue can be helpful and easy. Take it one treatment at a time before introducing too many changes at once. Take a deeper look at your skin when the seasons or your environment changes.

Trust me when I say your skin tells you what it needs. When you open up your observations, you'll be on the fast track to keeping your face in check when it's time for your wedding closeups!

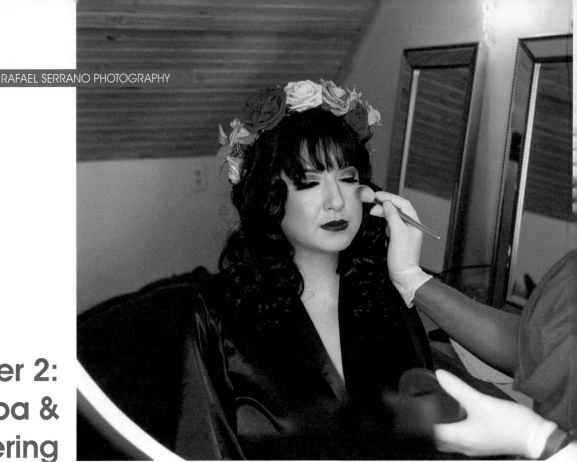
RAFAEL SERRANO PHOTOGRAPHY

Chapter 2: Medspa & Pampering

It's your wedding day preparation! That means it's time to treat yourself! This particular investment in your look will have you saying thank you for years into your marriage. Wink wink!

If you are looking to take your skincare to the next level, there are skin specialists that will take you there! A facial is one of the best ways to care for your skin. Seeking additional assistance from a professional dermatologist or esthetician can be just what brings out the beauty of your skin! Having a professional facial and advanced anti-aging treatments can be a relaxing and instant fix to concerns that a specialist can deliver. At the same time, you relax and hand it over to a trained professional.

A little maintenance now will save a lot of maintenance later! A facial can be viewed as a deeper evaluation of what concerns your skin can develop, followed by an essential treatment wedding treatment plan to keep your skin healthy and glowing.

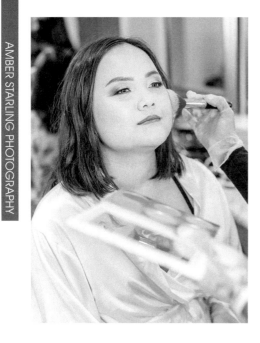

AMBER STARLING PHOTOGRAPHY

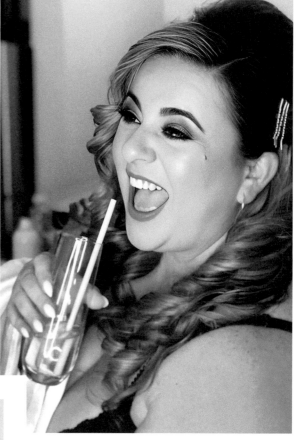

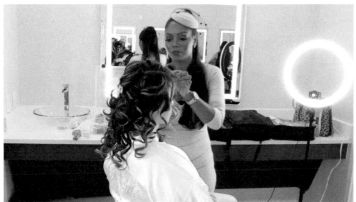

ON D SCENE PHOTO AND VIDEO

Skin care professionals typically recommend having a facial every 4-6 weeks on average, depending on the concerns to be addressed. Having one recommended more or less would be based on the professional advice of the administering professional. An evaluation followed by a treatment plan can assist you in your everyday skincare routine we addressed earlier and deeply treat the occasional flare-ups hormones leave our skin with. You can think of it as a deep cleaning treatment to back up your daily maintenance.

Say sayonara to that dead weight… literally! A treatment that virtually dissolves and lifts away problematic discoloration, softens expression lines, and increases cell turnover are results a professional-level exfoliating peel can deliver. Have you ever looked into the mirror or a picture and thought, "Wow, I look tired!?" Taking a moment to revive tired skin and relax could be an instant pick-up to brighten your appearance.

No pain, no gain, they say! Suppose a little pain never bothered you, and you're looking forward to a more aggressive approach to getting rid of visible age signs that have a natural finish. In that case, you can talk to your cosmetic dermatologist about what would be recommended for a week to reverse the signs of aging. As always, risks are involved, and you must outway the pros and cons with a professional before making a decision that impacts your appearance. Choosing a minimally invasive procedure, such as peels and temporary injectables, can provide more aggressive correction for more mature brides.

A skin treatment plan before your big day will make your skin look amazing and is a healthy habit to make a part of your routine. Healthy skin will not only make your makeup look more smooth and flawless, but it helps it perform longer and resist premature degradation caused by having oil-filled pores, dry skin texture, or crease lines from dehydrated skin. Since photos last a lifetime, diving deeply into skin health is a must!

Chapter 3: Choosing a Makeup Style

Now that we've covered skincare basics, we can jump right into your glam goals. One thing that will make your makeup selection process a breeze is to narrow down specifics of likes and dislikes. Starting from a basic list will help prepare you for what to include in your perfect wedding day look! From my industry experience, I've found that most brides either fall into 3 categories of makeup. Those consist of natural and clean, soft glam, and full glam.

You'll need to familiarize yourself with different levels of makeup before a bridal makeup trial. If you are familiar with having a professional makeup service, you can take a deep breath. You'll know half of what to expect. Seeing yourself dolled up into a studio-level transformation can be a bit overwhelming for those that have never seen themselves in professionally styled makeup.

Now comes the fun part! To further analyze what levels of makeup you'd be best wearing, you'll need to consider what you normally wear on a daily basis. Going for gorgeous is a definite must, but too much of a good thing may overwhelm you. Makeup harnesses the power to change your mood and affect your emotions, so you'll want to be mindful of the intensity. The last thing you'll want is to feel insecure about your appearance when you're the center of attention. Makeup is designed to define, empower and uplift! Hence, it shouldn't make you feel awkward and self-conscious.

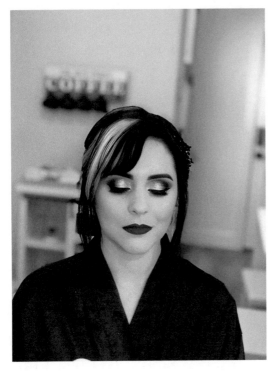

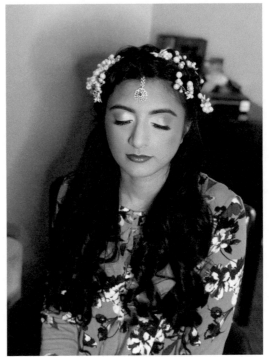

Ultimately, you should have a balanced look coordinated with your personal style, your wedding theme, the location, the season, and the time of your ceremony and reception.

To further analyze your personal style and tastes in makeup, let's dive into different categories that may help you determine where you fall. Be sure to tally up your score at the end to reveal which of the 3 makeup styles best suits your preferences!

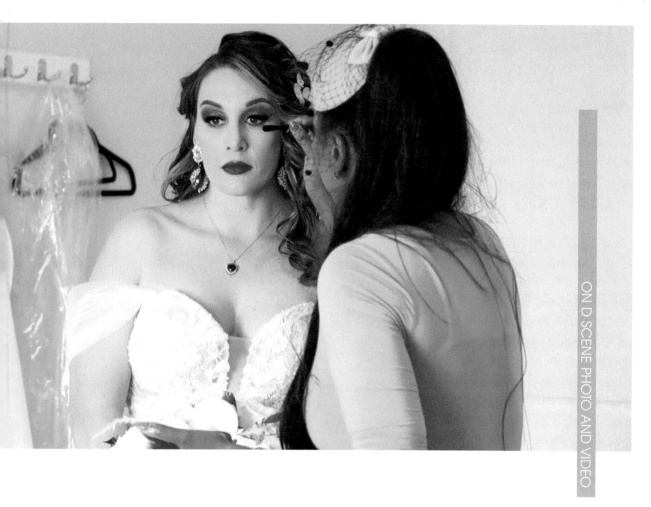

ON D SCENE PHOTO AND VIDEO

Foundation Coverage

Unbeknownst to most, foundation is formulated in different levels of opacity. You can find that most come in either light, medium, or full coverage. When you think about bb, cc cream, or tinted moisturizer, these tend to be more skin-like and have a thinner consistency. They fit into light coverage. It can be considered medium coverage when your skin is evenly covered in a way that balances out redness and slight color imbalances. Lastly, suppose you have active blemishes, scaring, dark spots, or otherwise want to look completely perfected and flawless. In that case, you can put yourself in the full coverage category.

- If you prefer light coverage, give yourself a 1.
- If you prefer medium coverage, give yourself a 2.
- If you prefer full coverage, give yourself a 3.

Foundation Type

You may have experienced slight anxiety when you go shopping for one foundation only to realize there are literally hundreds of different types. For your base to stay in place and look flawless, having a good understanding of your skin and how it handles the types is vital. Although there are many new creations every day, foundation can be broken down into liquid, airbrush, cream, or powder.

Your beauty professional should ask you what type of skin you have to determine which formula has the best outcome. A professional makeup artist is trained to modify the foundation properties by adjusting the foundation with cosmetic additives such as illuminators or thinners. For instance, mixing a liquid illuminator with a matte foundation to have a luminous finish rather than matte could be suitable for someone with combination skin, but skin wants a glowing look. It stays controlled as it has an added reflection while not making it more emollient. It is a suitable choice rather than applying a cream base foundation as a cream on oily skin would break down easily in the oily zones and look greasy in photos after a short time.

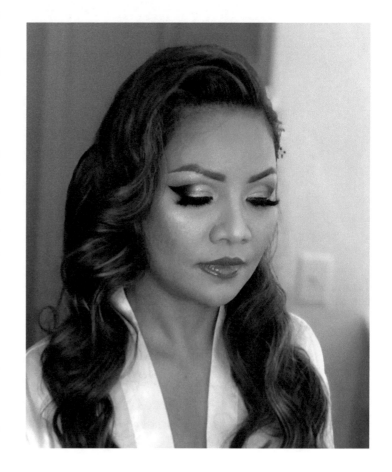

Cream foundation is a great choice for dry skin types. It can soften rough and scaly skin surfaces and feels nourishing. This would be a great choice if you want more coverage and a velvety finish! I would not recommend cream for someone concerned about looking heavy or creasing into fine lines and wrinkles. The thicker nature of the product needs to be set adequately to prevent transfer which adds more weight to the product and its look. Someone who loves full coverage would be in love with it, while someone who desires a lightweight natural look would be terrified! With that said, a cream can also be thinned out by mixing a cosmetic thinner. Your makeup artist can modify the creaminess and adjust the level of coverage easily.

If you are interested in a lightweight makeup finish, a foundation powder may be a suitable option. Keep in mind that corrections such as under-eye hollows and blemishes should be attended to before it is finished with a medium to full coverage face powder for a complete and balanced outcome. Some popular choices are mineral powers, sheer compact powders, and foundation powders.

Liquid is a popular choice due to its layering ability for more coverage and its flexibility in creating a fresh, lightweight finish and long-wear ability. By recognizing its benefits, you can understand what it aims to accomplish. It has many benefits of being hydrating, mattifying, or long wear, depending on the formula.

Airbrushed makeup is the go-to for the most flawless resurfacing effect. Contrary to its thin consistency, airbrush is so concentrated that it doesn't need to be piled on too heavily to provide flawless coverage. A small amount can be used for a lightweight finish over corrections or full coverage by adding thin layers. It may be thin, but it is powerful! Someone who likes a ceramic smooth filter finish would be thrilled to have this finish.

- Suppose you prefer a look closest to your skin and offers undetectability. In that case, you'd be comfortable with liquid or foundation powder types of finishes, so choose 1.
- If you're looking for a photo-ready look that feels comfortable and looks flawless and slightly transforming, you may find liquid or cream is a suitable choice, so choose 2.
- Suppose you are a fan of the most flawless look with all imperfections concealed and a finish so smooth it has a filter-like surreal finish. In that case, you'd be perfectly matched to cream or Airbrushed, so give yourself a 3.

Color Palette

The colors you choose in your makeup should align with your wedding colors. It doesn't need to be the exact shade of each but rather be in the same family of colors and temperatures and

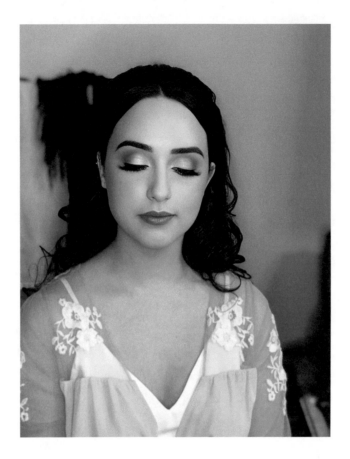

be complementary to each other. For example, a peachy combination is flattering with oranges, corals, and reds. Choosing a red lip will be a great choice if you have lots of greenery since red and green are complementary colors.

It will be worthwhile to consider the different types of color schemes: monochromatic, complementary, and analogous, and their placement on the color wheel. They are commonly used in color combinations for beauty as well as floral, decor, and fashion.

- If you prefer fresh neutral skin tones and minimal color, give yourself a 1.
- If you prefer earth-tone shades with a hint of color in the mix, give yourself a 2.
- If you prefer bold, true colors that make a statement, give yourself a 3

Color Intensity

Color has the possibility of altering the way you feel. Have you ever walked into a dark room and felt like your energy dropped, conversations became more direct, or your mood became serious? Being intune with certain colors and their intensity can positively impact your mood.

Often, the time of the ceremony weighs heavily on the decision to amplify the amount of intensity in makeup. Other times, it's the theme of the wedding and season in the year.

If your ceremony and reception are in daytime hours, in spring or summer, and in a garden of florals, going for a fresh, romantic, airy, or poppy look would be fitting. Suppose you plan for a fall celebration with the season's rich colors, and it's an evening affair. In that case, you may consider a look incorporating deep berries, plums, or rusty shades with a smoky touch to your eyes, which exudes sophistication, mystery, and strength.

A general rule of thumb is if it is daytime to keep it light and fresh and nighttime to turn up the glam, add more color and a sultry finish.

While rules are a great foundation to consider, rules are made to be broken if you want to take elements from either side and make them your own. After all, artistry is an expression of creativity and freedom. Staying within the rules may give you more comfort and stability if you are more strategic and formal.

- If you prefer simplicity, minimalism, muted colors, or pastels, give yourself a 1.
- If you prefer your best features to be amplified, can't go a day with eyeliner, and are not afraid to use a little color to coordinate your makeup to your outfit, choose 2.
- If you're into a sultry appeal, you intend to captivate onlookers with full-on color saturation, or vibrant colors make you feel alive, choose 3.

Lashes

One fancy way to magnify your eyes and help them look brighter and more beautiful is by doubling the lashes. With a long history in women's beauty, false lashes are in high demand. Hence, they can make a world of difference in professional photos! You can think of lashes as an accessory to your eyes. They are a very popular choice when taking photographs because they magnify your eyes. You can not see your natural lashes too well in a far-away photograph. Lashes help make them more flirty and visible. In a professional photography setting, makeup is applied with more contrast and color so that the amount of flash and light sources don't wash out colors excessively and your features stay properly defined.

Whether you are adding in a few clusters to fill spareness, are a regular customer at the lash extension salon, or enjoy wearing daily disposable lashes to complement your everyday look, considering lashes on your wedding day will make your eyes look more highlighted, emphasized, and flirty!

- If you are new to lashes and want to try them out for the first time, would like to wear glasses, like a simple, understated touch, choose 1.
- If you are looking for a romantic, flirty finish that looks soft and glamorous with visible and eye-catching lashes, choose 2.
- If you enjoy making a statement with your eyes, wear lashes as a part of your daily look, and are no stranger to a full fluffy finish, choose 3.

Skin Finish

The overall appearance of the face is mostly selected according to personal preference for most. When having professional pictures taken, your beauty professional should balance your skin finish according to different factors: current trends, age, skin type, whether you will be in a natural light studio, indoor or outdoor, the season, or you are having an evening event where high flash photography will be used.

To simplify skin finish options, you need to determine what you like most about how your skin looks. Generally, it's either glowing, matte, or satin, which is between the two. Matte has no shine and has a powdered finish, glowing has a luminous, dewy look, and satin has a balanced skin-like appearance.

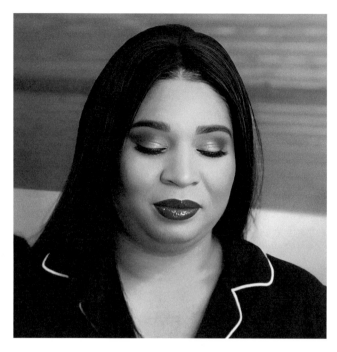

When choosing a skin finish, it is important to consider the time of year and the setting where you'll take photos. If you'll be outside in the heat, have oily skin, and be indoors in a flash-lit studio setting, it will be a wise choice to lean into a matte or satin finish. If it is a cold season or your skin type is dry or mature, opting for a luminous finish will give you a hydrated and fresh appearance.

- If you desire a clean, no-shine finish, choose 1
- If you want your face to have a natural appeal with some highlighting, choose 2.
- If you live for a glowing, glossy finish, choose 3.

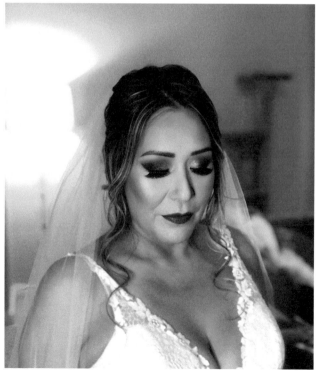

Eye Focus

If you've heard the saying, "Eyes are the windows to the soul," you may understand the effect eyes have on the entire face. With eyes being a focus feature, they really set the mood of the makeup! To pick the appropriate level of eye makeup that compliments your wedding theme, you should consider the intensity levels of the following three:

- eyeshadow
- eyeliner choices
- brow style

If most of your wedding activities are in the daytime, opting for an airy, soft look would be ideal. A matte finish with softer eyeshadow shading would be a great choice to keep things fresh. On the other hand, if your ceremony has a regal theme and your accessories are glitzy and sparkle, opting for a similar metallic finish and a smokey touch on your eyes would be fitting.

Using eyeliner will frame your eyes and will help them appear more defined. Your eye shape will also have a lot of weight in the selection. Choosing the best technique to highlight your particular eye shape should be considered.

More large prominent eyes benefit from full-liner techniques. Line the top and bottom lash line and the tight-lining technique that fills in the space behind the eyelashes work well. Someone with a larger eye may find that the framing look of fully lining balances the size of their eyes with other features of their face. Applying too little may not have an exciting effect.

Someone with a small or hooded eye shape should use caution to avoid over-lining. To prevent the eyes from looking even smaller, or worse, having a beady appearance, using a blended softer liner look or a no eyeliner technique would be suitable. Having a brighter bottom waterline may assist in making them appear larger. This can be achieved using beige or white eyeliner to finish the waterline.

Using a winged eyeliner look seems to be an everlasting trend. This dramatically transforms the eyes to look more alluring and have a seductive gaze. When this style is used, it can make the eyes appear more almond-shaped and wider. Trying different angles of the wing can give you an idea of which best fits your eye. A winged liner that is applied more straight would be good if they normally experience a line distortion from the crease overlapping at the end of the eye. A more upward angle creates a lifting effect and would be great for uplifting tired or downturned eyes.

Caution should be used if your eyes have a low or hooded crease or are wide set. Typically, in these cases, applying the eyeliner more upward angled and blending the hard edge smooth to create a shadowy wing instead of a hard line avoids line distortion. It also lifts the eyes upward instead of drawing them more lengthwise to the sides of the face.

Brows are a feature of the face that changes drastically between fashion trends. In the past, celebrities' and models' style choices have influenced beauty trends. They've ranged from a pencil-thin line to fluffy and natural! Since brows can completely set the mood of the entire look, they should not be forgotten. Exaggerated trends are not recommended for bridal makeup as it dates your photos. Have you ever looked back at old photos just to find yourselves cringing at styles you thought were amazing at the time? Bridal makeup should exude a timeless beauty appeal to appreciate for years to come.

By ensuring that your eyebrows are properly groomed, you'll be doing your beauty professional a favor as well as your photos. Taking a trip to have them trimmed, shaped, and tinted, if necessary, will ensure no unruly, discolored, or overgrown arches ruin your photo closeups!

Going to a professional brow expert is a great decision. They are trained to create the most flattering and balanced shapes for different eye and face shapes. Having your brows groomed a week prior should have them ready just in time for your big day.

To avoid hair removal mishaps, being aware of any medicine or topical face products should be researched for contraindications. Pregnancy, sunburns, facial treatments, using any products or medicines for controlling acne, and anti-aging skin care can make the skin more susceptible to getting damaged by hot wax. Far too many people are victims of burns and skin lifting by not being aware of this. When in doubt, ask an esthetician what the best options are. You certainly don't want to end up with scarring before your wedding day!

- If you prefer a clean matte eye look with minimal liner and natural brows, choose 1.
- If you prefer a shimmery finish with eyeliner that has an alluring defining appeal with naturally defined brows, choose 2.
- If you prefer a fully lined eye, a sultry smokey finish with a statement brow, choose 3.

Lip Focus

Lips are another focus feature that makes the entire look come together. The intensity should be balanced with the eyes and cheeks to have a harmonious effect. When you are speaking to your guests, they, of course, will adore all of you. But when engaging in direct conversation, many people focus on the mouth. Since many brides opt for different tones of white and ivory, lips can brighten up the face and add much-needed color, so you aren't washed out. Your lips may be the center of attention when speaking. To ensure lips properly define your look and stay in place, you should consider the shape of your lips, lip habits, color selection, and finish.

The shape of your lips can be more symmetrical and fuller with a little tweaking. Lip liner has been used now for about 100 years. Although it hasn't been around more than lipstick, it is an equally important tool for delivering a perfectly balanced and pretty pout. Lip liner has evolved into many uses. But you will find it useful in preventing feathering, emphasizing your Cupid's bow, and creating fuller and more even lips.

One of the favorite pieces of advice I give brides to prepare them for a day of looking beautiful is, "Remember to eat pretty!"

Along with that, drinking pretty and kissing pretty should mentally follow. This may seem new to you if you have never had to keep lipstick on for more than 2 hours, but it will come in handy for looking polished for all those photos to come. You must be aware of your lip movements and daily habits. Pay close attention to how you eat, wipe your mouth after eating, drink out of a glass, rub your lips back and forth or lick your lips constantly, and kiss your partner.

When you eat, try to minimize the amount of outer lip contact by choosing smaller bites, placing food carefully into the mouth, and using a combination of your tongue, teeth, and the inner part of your lips to slide it off. When you take a drink, you should try to find the same place on the rim of your glass. If you can place the rim of the glass further onto the lip, this would prevent constant lipstick transfer. A good method to remember is to find your lipstick mark and give yourself a kiss. Of course, theoretically! You certainly don't want to go around kissing cups.

If you have noticed that your lipstick doesn't last long even after trying longwear formulas, you may have a habit of rubbing your lips together or licking them. Both should be eliminated as the constant friction breaks down lipstick, allowing it to smudge or peel away easily, and licking your lips will have you ingesting it.

Not kissing your partner is impossible on the big day! I wouldn't want anyone to feel constricted on such a special occasion celebrating love. Learning to kiss pretty will probably be the most fun practice out of all that was mentioned. Most notably, aiming for a perfect peck on the lips throughout your photoshoot and celebrations is ideal. Kissing guests' cheeks should be done through the infamous cheek kiss, in which you greet guests by touching cheeks and mimicking a kiss with an audible kiss sound. Remember to kiss the air, not the actual cheek.

Practice makes perfect, and it will be hard at first to modify some of these actions to keep your lipstick from wearing away prematurely, but the hard work will pay off in the long run.

In most cases, lipstick for a wedding is not permanent. Paying close attention to the lip finish may help you decide which is best, considering all your habits. Lipstick with a matte finish generally transfers less, while glossed lips tend to wear down and smudge more easily. If you are set on a rich color and have concerns about lipstick transferring on your loved ones, it would be best to keep it matte. Suppose your favorite lipstick is creamy and does not dry down matte. In that case, an industry secret is to set your lips with a transparent powder to make them matte and less transferable. If you can not live without a glossy finish, you may want to lean into natural, softer colors that will not be as noticeable when exchanging kisses. If you want the best of both worlds, there are two-step lip products in which the color is applied. It sets completely then clear gloss is applied on top. The gloss can be refreshed throughout the day to keep it shiny, while the color adheres to the lips for all-day wear.

Now that we've nailed down some behavior modifications that assist in keeping your lips pretty, we can move into color selection. Your lip intensity should be balanced with your eyes. If your eyes are dramatic, a soft lip is ideal. If your eyes and overall makeup are on the softer side, a statement lip would be great!

Mentioning your wedding colors to your beauty professional is vital to ensuring your makeup colors match and coordinate well. After all, your bouquet is held close to your face and shouldn't clash. Some good tricks for a great lip choice include coordinating it with your eyes or cheeks color. For example, if one of your wedding colors is purple, choosing a plum or mauve would be complementary. If your eyeshadows are neutral earth tones, you should lean into either a variation of one of your wedding colors or opt for a neutral pink nude. For example, if your wedding is in the spring and your color palette has blue and green tones, choosing a rich coral lipstick would be complementary.

- If you prefer a natural lip shape and soft lip colors, and tend to not be bothered by behavioral modifications for enhancing lip wear, choose 1.
- If you prefer your lips to be balanced out by incorporating natural lip lining, don't mind either a matte or glossy lip finish, and don't mind a bit of fading because you can refresh it later, choose 2.

- If you prefer to overline your lips for a juicy pout, don't mind achieving all the steps required to keep your lips perfect, and wouldn't blink at purchasing a two-step lipstick to lock on your lips all day, choose 3.

Contour and Blush Level

Adding depth, highlight, and color to the face is vital to keep makeup looking dimensional. Without it, the wearer would appear pale, sick, washed out, and ghostly in photos. Since brides mostly opt for light-colored gowns, it's best to add a higher level of shading and color to the face. This will ensure the brides show up in photographs properly and do not get washed out by the amount of lightness of the dress. Bridal makeup should put more of an emphasis on rosy cheeks and contours for that extra special bridal touch!

The dimension level should be addressed differently depending on age and skin tone factors. If a bride is more mature, adding more blush than contour would be a better balance. As we age, the amount of natural healthy color in the cheeks disappears. Adding a more rosy cheek helps by giving the bride a more youthful glow. Excessive contour should be avoided in mature brides as this will bring more attention to the loss of volume in the cheeks and face and make them appear gaunt.

Contrary to popular belief, deep complexions need blush as well. All skin tones benefit from blush and contouring as it balances the color in the makeup and defines your best features! The cheek color and lipstick should be in the same color family and match the theme of the wedding colors. If no blush were applied, it would cause a disconnect in the look and make it appear like something is missing.

The contrast level with blush and contouring can be personal to each bride. Generally, a smaller amount of blush is applied for a more soft look, and more is applied for a more glamorous finish.

Factors such as having your ceremony inside or outside may weigh in on the decision to use cream or powder products. Real natural sunlight is very good at magnifying the amount of makeup applied. Opting for lightweight face makeup would be best if you are getting married outside. Layers of creamy makeup can appear and feel heavy under the beaming sunlight and have a higher chance of creasing from squinting and, unfortunately, smearing and getting oily from factors such as heat from the sun.

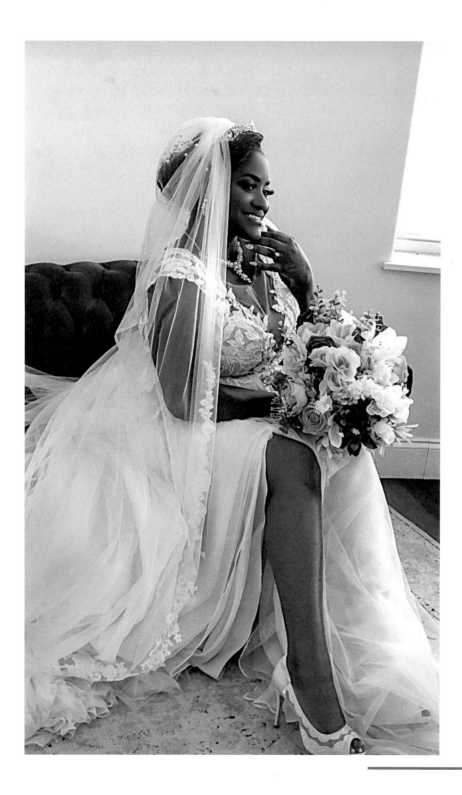

- If you prefer a soft level of blush and contour, choose 1.
- If you prefer your face to be balanced with a studio level of contouring and rosy cheeks, choose 2.
- If you prefer a sculpted contour that may emphasize your best features, minimize undesired features such as chin fatty tissue or face roundness, and enjoy blushed cheeks, choose 3.

Now that you've learned about the different types of makeup styles and components of each category, please take a moment to tally up your score to reveal your makeup style preference below:

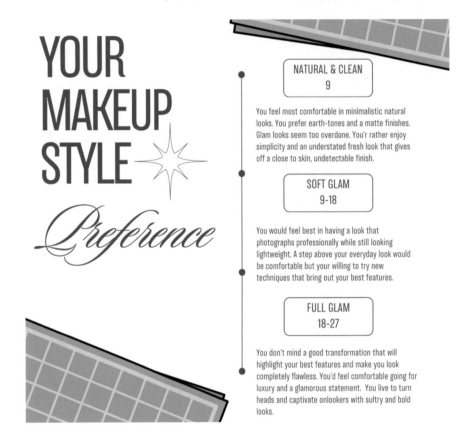

YOUR MAKEUP STYLE *Preference*

NATURAL & CLEAN
9

You feel most comfortable in minimalistic natural looks. You prefer earth-tones and a matte finishes. Glam looks seem too overdone. You'r rather enjoy simplicity and an understated fresh look that gives off a close to skin, undetectable finish.

SOFT GLAM
9-18

You would feel best in having a look that photographs professionally while still looking lightweight. A step above your everyday look would be comfortable but your willing to try new techniques that bring out your best features.

FULL GLAM
18-27

You don't mind a good transformation that will highlight your best features and make you look completely flawless. You'd feel comfortable going for luxury and a glamorous statement. You live to turn heads and captivate onlookers with sultry and bold looks.

Choosing a makeup style according to your comfort level is important to ensure you feel gorgeous and not overwhelmed. Next to your preferences should be those of your bridesmaids and mother.

A very popular question among many brides is how the bridal party's makeup should look. It is completely your choice! Remember that this is your wedding, and you will most likely invest significant time and money in this grand celebration. Your bridal party will be in most of your professional photos and videos. Many of the shots taken of you will include your bridal party partaking in the process.

After you have your look narrowed down, it's time to shift your focus on how they should look. Having professional hair stylists and makeup artists can outright raise the level of class and professionalism in your photos. One of my favorite sayings is, "If you're having professional photos taken, your hair and makeup should be professionally styled."

Since your wedding day photos will be a timeless representation of your love for years to come, you should consider what will be framed and on display to look at... for eternity! This it's not just one day; it will be memories of a lifetime.

Factoring in your budget will be the first step. You'll need to see what your budget will allow you to cover. It's important to know that the prices of bridal specialists are usually higher than regular services. It is a top-tier beauty industry category, and only very experienced and skilled artists can work in bridal. Years of experience, training, and administration are factored into ensuring your experience is high quality and runs smoothly and professionally.

Since money doesn't flow the same for everyone, some popular options brides give their bridal party participants are the following:

- Paying for both hair and makeup.
- Paying for one service and having them choose hair or makeup.
- Paying for one service as a half-and-half deal, then having them cover the other half.

After considering what you'd like to invest in, you can move to styling choices. You are the main attraction and reason for the celebration! This means that your bridesmaids should be dialed down so you can take center stage. If you go back to your comfort level with makeup, bridesmaids should match this level or be a notch under.

For example, if you choose light and fresh, everyone else needs to be light and fresh. If you choose full glam, everyone needs to be full glam, a soft version of your style, or natural beauty makeup. It's popular for brides to have their bridesmaids' makeup incorporate wedding colors. Having their eyeshadow incorporate one of your wedding colors would be complementary.

Moms have a category of their own when it comes to hair and makeup. Generally, mothers should not choose something that is completely out of their traditional look for dressy events. Often, they would feel uncomfortable doing this initially. Since they typically have their own dress color aside from the bridesmaids, their makeup should complement their style preferences and what they wear.

Chapter 4: Age-appropriate Makeup

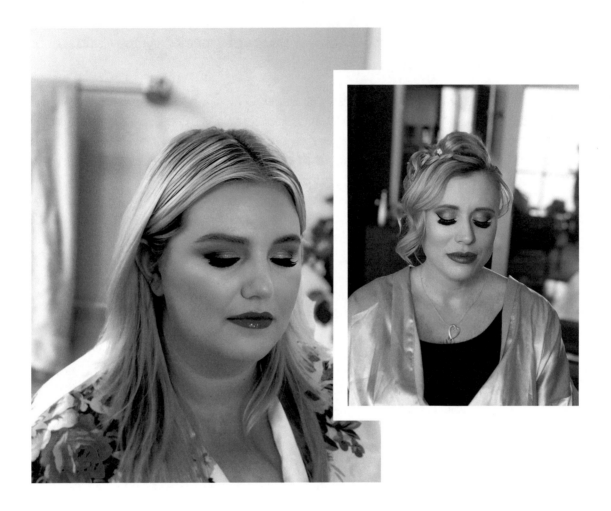

Have you ever looked in your makeup storage and found something you haven't seen in years? As women, I think we can all relate to buying makeup, using it for a while, and then completely forgetting about it. You may want to keep makeup around for sentimental reasons, but you should assess if the particular makeup style is serving you properly.

Application methods and types of makeup looks change constantly. In addition to that, we are also changing with age. It is important to ensure that your current techniques are up to date according to what is most flattering for your age group.

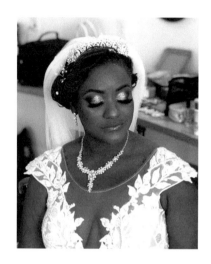

For brides in their 20s, trends may call out to you like a moth to a flame! Although you may be tempted to wear the hottest trends, keep in mind that bridal makeup is best when it exudes a timeless appeal. While incorporating small hints here and there is perfect for adding a boldness and a personal touch, going for extreme trends will severely date your photos in the future. Adding fun touches to your makeup, such as a brighter poppy lip color, or shimmery and even glitter finishes,

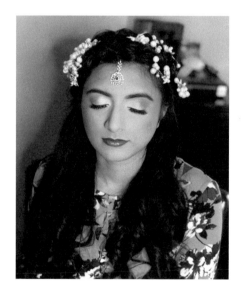

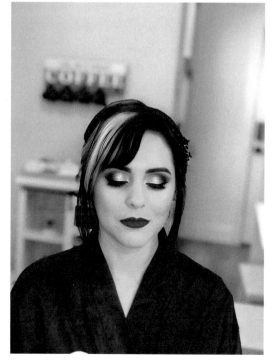

will keep your look youthful and hip. Products that are either oil-free or oil-controlling would be ideal since younger brides tend to have more concerns with oily skin.

Choosing a classic beauty look would be flattering if you are in your 30s or 40s. By this time, you may notice adding more blush to your cheeks in a rounder application is more flattering than contouring blush methods. Having the focus of blush on your apples will add a more plump, youthful look. More richness on the cheeks and lips and a focus on brightening the under eyes will diminish the look of hollowness and dark circles. At this time in your life, you may notice the effects of aging begin to appear in the form of expression lines. It is important to not use heavy layers of makeup around these areas to avoid creases. A good trick is to build in thin layers to build up to the desired result, blot with a sponge to blend smoothly, and set with a lightweight translucent powder, paying close attention to the areas where you move your face the most.

Mature brides love to have a fresh, glowing appearance! Products that simulate a more luminous look, such as a liquid illuminator, will do wonders for maintaining the glow for hours. Since mature skin tends to be on the drier side, mixing a liquid illuminator in with your skincare or foundation will allow the look to stay longer. The nourishing properties of moisturizers tend

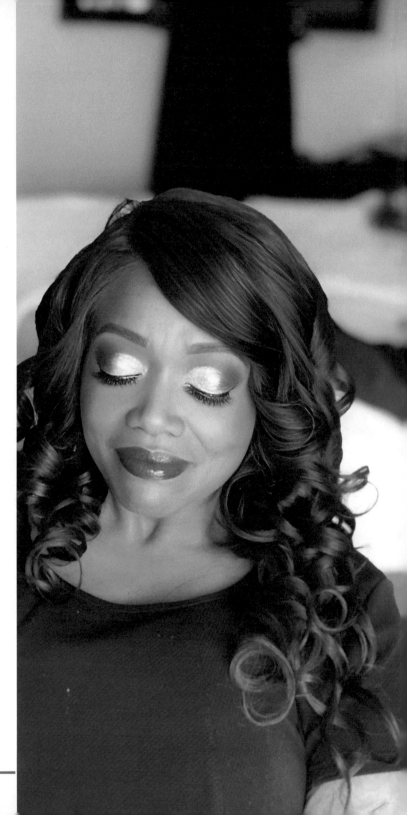

to absorb more quickly on mature skin, so it is helpful to add a layer of cosmetics that have a reflective nature.

Thinner is better when it comes to coverage on aging skin. The fresher and more lightweight your face looks, the more it will look youthful over the length of the wedding festivities. At this time in life, color correction may be necessary for dark marks and covering sun damage. Heavy creams and powders should be avoided in the expression areas as they have a greater tendency to crease. Using finely milled translucent powder on the areas that furrow easily is essential. Also, using the powder only on those places while keeping the cheeks unset would be best for keeping the glow. Cream or gel blush will add to the freshness.

A vital tip to remember for a mature bride is to avoid harshness. The use of heavy and sharp eyeliner will make the eyes appear smaller. Softly blended eyeliner is more flattering. Since lips are a focus feature, dark lipstick should be avoided due to its shrinking nature. Lips tend to get smaller with time so using light-colored lipstick on lips that have been slightly overdrawn helps to liven up the face.

Chapter 5: Day-of Essentials

Picture this; it is one of the most special moments of your life! You've hired the best professionals you could find and had a fantastic time getting ready with your best friends. You've had your first look photos and had the best, most memorable experience tying the knot with your significant other. Now, it's time to party! Then you slip into your dressing room for a bathroom break to look at the newly married woman you've become. You glance in the mirror and notice… tear marks down your cheeks, a lash corner lifting, your skin has become oily, your lips have been kissed away, and your uncle did get his watch caught in your hair on that hug. Also, some curls have been pulled from your chignon!

Although all this sounds like a living nightmare, it's all relative to situations that happen at weddings. One of the best things you can do is prepare yourself for the unexpected. There are essential items that you do not want to leave without! Be sure to pack your bag with these items to help you stay polished from the ceremony to the last toast.

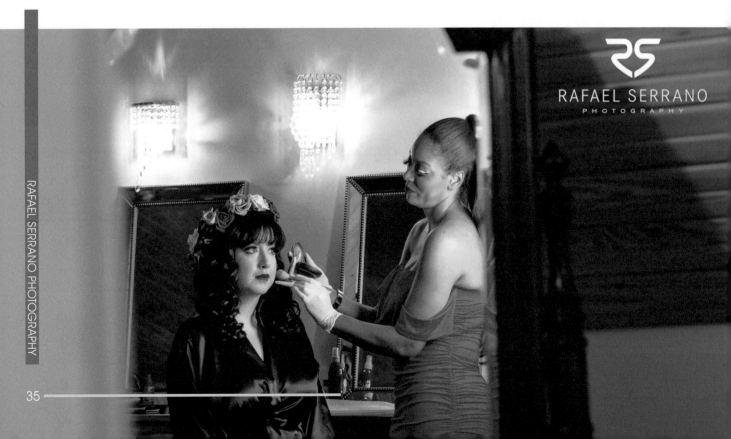

RAFAEL SERRANO PHOTOGRAPHY

Makeup Touch-up Essentials:

1. Clear eyelash adhesive
   - With so many happy tears involved, having this product to tack down lifting corners will be a lifesaver.
2. Concealer
   - Using this product as a correcting tool is ideal for patching face makeup. Underneath the eyes can be especially important to refresh from tearing. Squinting from the bright sun or smiling can break down and crease the under eye. A small dab will go a long way to keeping it fresh.
3. Mascara
   - Applying a fresh coat of mascara to lashes after crying will lift drooping lashes and make eyes appear awake.
4. Eyeliner
   - Using a little extra liner can really take your daytime look to a more dramatic touch for an evening reception.
5. Lipstick
   - Kissing will most definitely be involved! If you find yourself licking your lips often or accidentally wiping them away after eating, having a backup tube will be handy for refreshing your look.
6. Lip gloss
   - Gloss looks amazing and glams up your look for photos. Unfortunately, it doesn't last as long as lipstick, so keeping it on hand will be handy for photo sessions with your guests.
7. Sheer powder in your skin color
   - Oily skin helps keep your skin youthful, but it should be avoided in photography, especially at night time. Flash photography makes it appear even more dramatic. Keeping your shine in check is key for a fresh and clean look at all times.
8. Blush
   - Blush tends to fade quickly with motion, heat, and perspiration. Having it on hand will prevent you from looking washed out.

9. Tissues
   - You can't predict a sneeze or when you will shed a tear. Remember to catch your tears with a tissue by blotting gently. Stopping them around the eye area can save your face from needing to be corrected.

10. Makeup wipes
    - Lipstick smudge across your chin from eating is the worst! Having wipes on hand makes fixing that easy. They also come in handy for blotting small makeup or food stains on clothes.

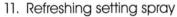

11. Refreshing setting spray
    - This is a must-have if you have dry skin. Refreshing your face after touching up your makeup will settle the powdery finish and make it look hydrated and fresher. It also comes in handy for calming nerves.

12. Mini mirror
    - Keeping this in your purse will allow you to see close up for small areas and make repairs.

13. Cotton swabs
    - This multi-purpose product can be amazing for cleaning up small smears, dabbing tears, or a cure for that little tickle sensation you get to scratch your face! It is important not to scratch or touch your face with your hands and fingers. This will avoid getting makeup on your dress. Fingers add oil to your face, making it shiny more quickly. Use cotton swabs gently as needed.

14. Straws
    - Before the ceremony and photos, these are useful for drinking. It works great for keeping your lipstick on.

15. Hand Fan
    - Nerves and anxiety can make you get overheated quickly. This can be used to cool yourself down and dry your face from perspiration, setting spray, and tears.

AMBER STARLING PHOTOGRAPHY

16. Tweezers
    - Sometimes it may seem like pesky facial hairs spring up overnight. This tool not only plucks out unwanted hair but also assists in steadying your hand while affixing false lashes.

Hair Essentials:

1. Comb
    - Use this to smooth down flyaways after spraying with hairspray.
2. Brush
    - Use this on a windy day or to remove tangles from extensions or unruly hair.
3. Bobby pins
    - You'll need to be sure you have an ample supply of these should there be the need for corrections to slipping-out curls and accidental bumps. They also come in handy for styling the hair half up if the hair around your face becomes bothersome.
4. Hairspray
    - Smoothing flyaways, recurling, and refinishing an updo with more is never a bad idea.
5. Hair ties
    - You may want to put your hair up in an easy updo later in the night. Perhaps your hair has sweated, and you'd rather have a clean bun than it to look messy. You can never go wrong with having a couple of these.
6. Hot tools
    - Having a blow dryer, curling iron, and flat iron to refresh fallen curls is a great way to maintain your look. Surely, there are days when your curls have lasted from morning to night. But with so much movement and commotion and possible unavoidable elements such as rain, humidity, and long exposure to outside heat, you can never be too prepared. If your curls don't stay well beyond a couple hours, it is vital that you bring hot tools.

Fashion Emergency Essentials:

1. Safety pins
    - These are necessary for some cultural traditions of fabric draping and also handy for clothing malfunctions.
2. Emergency sewing kit

- With nervous hands buttoning and zipping up garments, accidents are bound to happen. Having a needle and thread handy is vital.

3. Lint roller
   - Neat and polished is the way to be for important celebrations. Ensure your pet's hair doesn't end up making you look unorderly.

4. Deodorant
   - With the nerves in full effort, the last thing you'd want to stress about is smelling bad. Nervous sweating is certainly common, so having a backup spray-on community deodorant is a must.

5. Small first aid kit
   - Whether it's small children being around or a clumsy mistake, you'll be relieved to have this little kit of wonders!

6. Handheld steamer
   - This is a great travel tool for special occasions. Since everyone's level of ironing and clothes care may not be up to par, ensure you have this for erasing those pesky wrinkles.

7. Tide stain removal pin
   - If you are a clumsy eater or have children in attendance, this is vital to erasing food and drink spillage from clothing.

8. Fashion tape
   - Use this to fix falling straps and low necklines that may accidentally overexpose.

9. Shoe grips and pads
   - New shoes are very pretty but can also cause pretty painful situations of rubbing against your foot, slipping off, or sliding around due to having a fresh sole. This can be quickly fixed by these easy additions.

10. Perfume
    - Because it's always a great idea to smell amazing.

11. Lotion
    - This could be easily forgotten with so many other things to grab before leaving. There's nothing worse than having itchy, dry skin when trying to look fabulous!

12. Feminine hygiene products
    - Need I say more?

Now that we've covered your day-of essentials and overviewed what to be prepared for, you should ask yourself if it is worth the stress to take care of yourself. Another thing to consider is the investment in all these products and the skill level required to execute many of them. Now ask, can you rely upon your bridal party to bring these items?

It's essential to consider your options to see that your wedding day goes as planned with as little stress as possible. If what you've just read seems like an overwhelming amount of duties to be in charge of, delegating it to a professional may be the best option. It may cost less to have a service provider take care of it.

From my professional experience of working hundreds of weddings, I have witnessed many events in which having these items could have made a world of difference. This is a great example of why my company offers couples touch-up and on-set styling services.

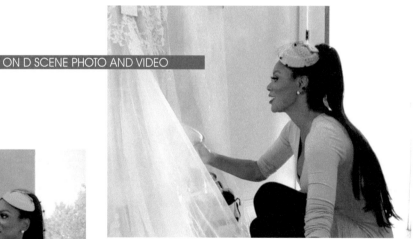

ON D SCENE PHOTO AND VIDEO

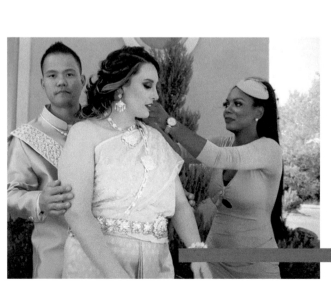

ON D SCENE PHOTO AND VIDEO

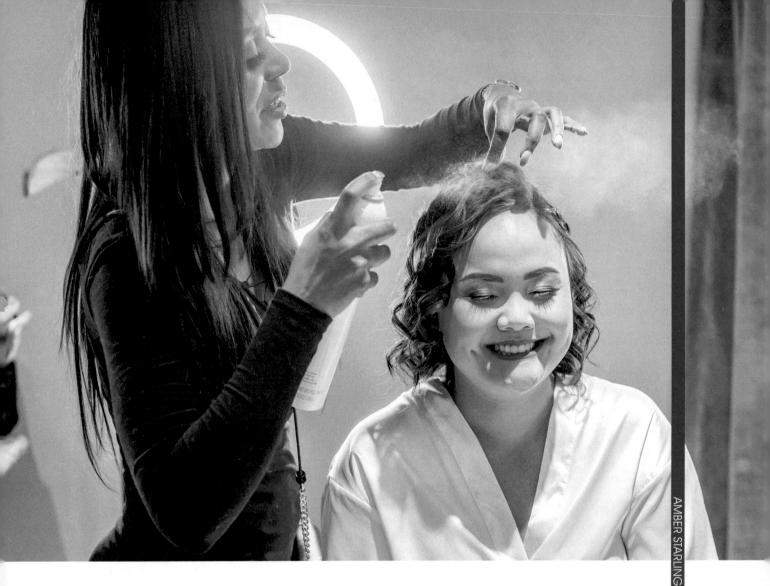

AMBER STARLING PHOTOGRAPHY

Chapter 6: Hair Care & Prep

Raise your hand if you want beautiful, healthy hair for your wedding day! To have the best hair results, you must investigate the current health of your hair and choose the best plan of action to ensure your hair is in the best shape to perform and look the way you want. The first step to analyzing your hair health is determining what it could benefit from.

Many factors make up different ways to take care of hair, including genetics and ethnic background. Since everyone's hair type has its own set of rules for maintenance, starting with the difficulties you may have encountered may be the easiest route.

Curly Hair

Curly hair can have a learning process that is unique to each person. One thing that all curly hair has in common is its tendency to become dry and frizzy. Luckily, there have been some major advances in curly hair products in the market. I can admit that having products made specifically for wearing natural curls have come a long way!

If you imagine hair like the roots of a tree, this will give a great visual of why hair becomes frizzy. The roots of a tree are constantly changing directions and growing in different directions in search of water. Likewise, hair lacking moisture tends to become frizzy and unruly due to its search for moisture in the air.

"One of the most important things to consider for curly hair is ensuring it stays hydrated."

Washing it too often or using the wrong type of shampoo and conditioner can cause dryness and tangles. Washing your hair and using a deep conditioner afterward is ideal. A good tip for detangling is to use a wide-toothed comb in the shower while your hair is saturated with conditioner.

While styling, apply cream and oil designed to hydrate and smooth curly hair. This is essential to keeping it healthy. Argan and coconut oil are my favorite oils for a bouncy, polished finish. Used as a finishing step, applying a small amount of oil will seal in your products, shine hair and soften the

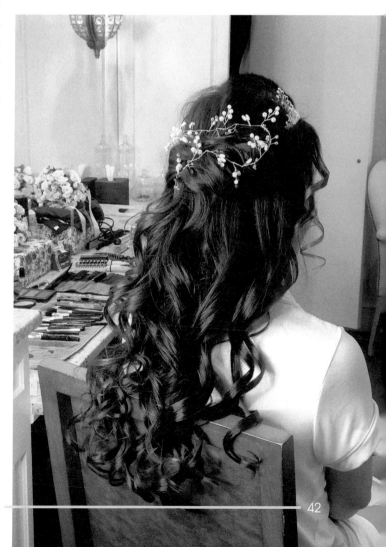

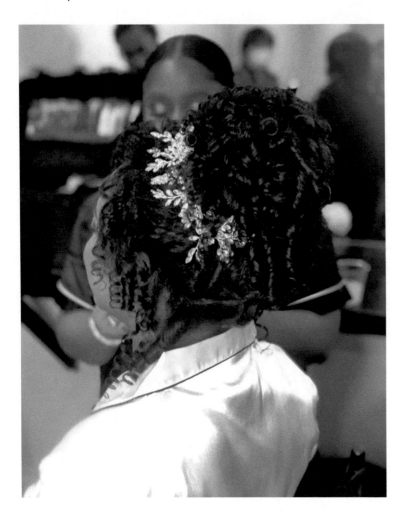

crunch of the styling products that are designed to hold.

Some of the most important methods of drying curly hair include using ample curling butter, cream, or leave-in conditioning treatment. This will prevent the hair from becoming a big poof when you want defined spirals and waves. Using a styling product that will hold the curl pattern, such as setting login or mousse designed for curly hair, will allow it to stay defined through moments of humidity, rain, and wind.

Since curly hair is more susceptible to brittleness and heat damage, always use heat-protectant products before applying heat, add moisture daily, and protect it at night by braiding, twisting, or putting it in a bun. If you want to go the extra mile, use a bonnet or scarf to protect your hair while sleeping.

One of the best secrets for creating a picture-worthy, naturally curly bridal hairstyle is having the stylist use a smaller curling wand and apply curls throughout the natural curls strands to create a more defined pattern.

These studio secrets will have everyone fooled and create the most fantastic curly look for your wedding day!

Oily and Imbalanced Hair and Scalp

Have you ever noticed that your roots are always flat, and your hair gets oily quickly? Or do you have a flaky, itchy scalp that is recurrent?

It's time to clarify your hair when you notice the following:

- Your roots are flat and oily even after a fresh shampoo
- Curls fall out quickly from the roots to midshaft and look limp
- Hair feels weighed down, and your conditioning products are no longer working the same
- You're losing more hair stands than usual
- Hair doesn't absorb hydrating products
- Hair feels rough and looks dull
- You have an itchy, flaky scalp

Rebalancing improves the hair in several ways that can enhance your style. A minor adjustment to your hair care routine is a very easy way to achieve proper pH levels. This way, you can go longer without washing your hair and rid your scalp of irritation.

Using a clarifying shampoo once a month will ease these ailments and can transform lifeless hair into bouncy and fresh strands. You can think of a clarifying shampoo as a beefed-up cleanser. It deeply cleanses by releasing the stubborn build-up of oil, dirt, and products. Due to its stripping nature, you should always follow up with a nourishing, deep conditioning treatment to replenish hydration. If you have color-treated hair, attention must be used to purchasing a product designed for colored hair.

To ensure your hair is prepped for your wedding day, start the clarification process at least 2 months before to fully understand how often it should be done. For some, once a month is perfect. For others, every two weeks is the sweet spot.

In addition to clarifying your hair, attention should be paid to using the correct hair products in your daily and weekly regimen. If your scalp is oily, choosing a balancing shampoo and conditioner combination on a regular basis will keep your hair looking its best. Choosing a lightweight and volumizing version of leave-in products will also assist.

On the other hand, if your scalp has recurrent flakes and itchiness, you may want to exfoliate it with a scrubbing comb while you wash your hair. There are also products on the market that have a granular consistency designed to break down dead skin cells and residue on the scalp's surface and properly balance the hydration levels. After a more strenuous cleansing treatment, always use a deep conditioner designed for your particular hair concern. You'll be rewarded with a scalp and hair that feels refreshed and rebalanced.

As mentioned above, it's best to start any new process of clarifying your hair and scalp at least two months prior to truly understand how often it should be performed and how your hair reacts to the products.

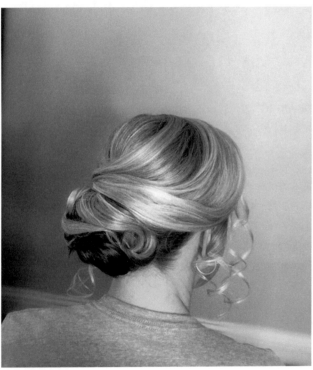

Processed and Unruly Hair

It would seem like these two go hand in hand. Having processed hake can sometimes lead to unmanageable, unruly hair and vice versa. If your hair is chemically processed with color, bleached, uses a straightening system, perms, or is texturized, it will likely need special care to ensure it remains healthy.

A very common concern with this hair type is dryness, dullness, and breaking. You must use products designed for what type of chemical treatment is done to prevent further damage. Next to investing in the proper hair care products is ensuring that you go to a professional hairstylist to manage your processing. Going cheap on your hair is never beneficial in the long run. Be sure to invest in high-quality products and listen to your hair stylist's treatment suggestions and how often you should be seen.

To help prep your hair to be healthy and manageable for your wedding day, start with regular trims to your ends as soon as possible. At least every 8-12 weeks should be considered. If your hair is heat styled often and gets damaged easily, going on the soonest end will allow your hair to stay ahead of those pesky split ends.

A deep conditioning treatment should be used consistently to keep unruly hair manageable. Deep conditioning is designed to repair damaged and weakened hair. It penetrates the hair more deeply than a traditional conditioner and supplies it with repairing, nourishing ingredients. Starting with one time a month would be a great place to start for most people. If you feel your hair gets very dry within a few weeks, it's time to do the process again.

For hair that is extremely damaged, you may need to start with every week until your hair can be repaired. There can always be too much of a good thing! If you begin to notice signs that your hair feels limp and has a mushy or gummy texture

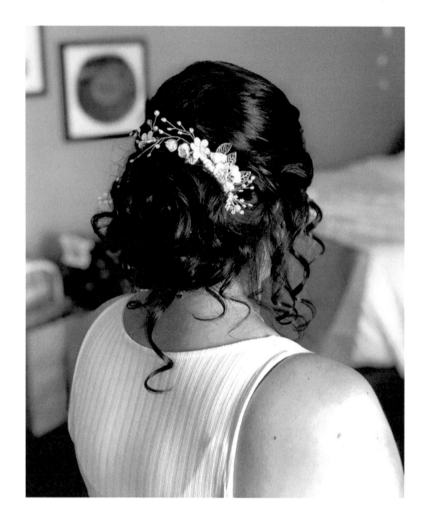

when wet, scaling back on the times you use the treatment should be made.

Any color processing, chemical straightening, and texture services should be completed at least weeks before your wedding. By this time, you should be comfortable with a stylist and have a solid understanding of the style direction. Appointments should be reserved well in advance to guarantee your time slot and preferred stylist. Although you may be tempted to try something new or chop it, this is not the time for big changes. Nine out of ten brides regret making a dramatic change after it's done!

Fiona Taylor

Since every bride wants hair that is healthy, shiny, and bouncy, incorporating a hair vitamin can ensure all the effort you put in pays off. A vitamin specially designed for hair may contain nutrients that boost and shine, help diminish hair loss, and stimulate hair follicles for growth and strength. By taking a hair vitamin, you are essentially treating your hair from the inside out. With anything great, you must spend the time. It takes about 3-6 months to truly see a difference if you take them religiously.

Now that you've learned the tricks you can do before the wedding day, it's time to talk about what to do to prepare it for your stylist on that special day. You should arrive at your hair appointment with completely dry and detangled hair. Arriving with damp hair is not good for heat styling. Your hair will be exposed to excessive heat and sizzle on the irons. It is also important to mention that blow drying will take additional time. But unfortunately, you'll not have a lot of time on your wedding day.

Hair that has been washed the day before will perform the best. Please note that any products you already apply that enhance your hair manageability should be applied before your appointment. These include a leave-in treatment, blow dry protectant, creams, or serums. Arriving with dry, frizzy hair is not ideal. Applying a volumizing mousse to your roots to mid-shaft before blow drying will allow for great lift.

Lastly, what to wear should be considered. I've seen plenty of brides need to cut out of their shirts due to not having the proper clothing. Taking off a tight-collared shirt will be difficult and may run the risk of ruining your hairstyling and smearing your makeup.

You should pack a comfortable camisole with shorts, a strappy nightgown, or a button-up shirt outfit. The first two should be worn under a robe. Having custom-printed or matching outfits for pictures is very popular. Not only does it make great getting-ready photos, but it also serves a great purpose of changing quickly into your wedding gown.

Chapter 7: Choosing a Hairstyle

Choosing a HairstyleIf you can relate to "having so many choices and not being able to choose one style," reading this chapter will give you peace of mind and a clear direction on choosing the most appropriate hairstyle for your wedding day.

One of the first things you've chosen is your overall theme. This will set the mood for many decorations throughout your wedding, including your beautiful look. Some popular themes include:

Bohemian- Draws inspiration from the '70s. Includes a relaxed and rustic style incorporating feathery plants, earthy tones, beading, macramé details, and outside settings.

Country/Barn- This theme is typically paired with its location of being on a farm and having an elegantly decorated barn for the ceremony or reception. Rustic details using wood, chalk-written signs, cowboy boots, and Mason jars make this theme feel homey and beautiful.

Nautical- A popular choice for destination, beach, or lake weddings. This style incorporates elements from the sea. Color tones such as navy blue and emerald green and coastal motifs paired with a classic undertone are essential.

Vintage Hollywood- Settings revolve around ornate decor, dripping luxury, chandeliers, crystals, and the color red. You'll be taken back in time to the 1920s-1940s.

Fantasy- If your favorite novel, period, or movie is the center of your inspiration, you'll find your theme picture-perfect as if it came straight out of a fictional storybook. Some popular concepts are Day of the Dead, Star Track, fairytale, Alice in Wonderland, Regency London Era, the Baroque time period, the Renaissance time period

Minimalist- Simple and understated is just enough for you. Limited but high-quality elements are considered. Often geometric shapes and metallics are selected.

Seasonal- Your wedding date may be close to a particular holiday. Popular choices are Christmas, New Year's, or Halloween. These holiday decorations will determine the entire vibe and mood.

Traditional- Very clean and timeless appeal with black and white colors. Details are not overdone or do not lean into fads or trends.

To make your look cohesive, consider a look that embraces the overall theme. Going with a look that doesn't fit your design elements will visibly clash. You must break down what hairstyle would be sensible if you were living in your particular theme setting. You'll be living in that dream world for an entire day!

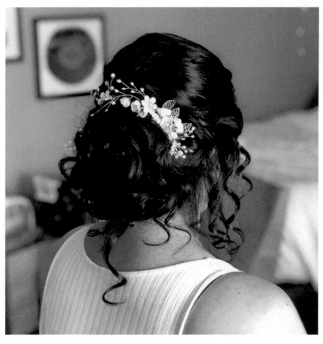

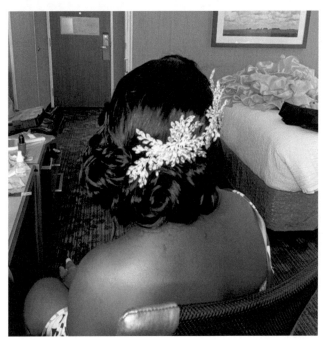

Generally, features of your theme can give you great inspiration for how you'd like your hair styled. Your hair should match the energy of the elements sounding it. Dress details such as the neckline, style, and fabric should be considered. Your gown may have a high or low neckline or include decorative details like a draping back. An updo will be a great choice if you want to show off the detail around the neckline. The last thing you will want is for your hair to get tangled in the decoration. A drawback to beaded neckline detail is that it risks strands of hair getting caught up in the design. Simply eliminate that situation with an updo!

If you have a strapless gown, wearing your hair half up will look feminine, soft, and classy while showing off the neckline. The warmth of your hair may come in handy for drafty moments and cooler days.

Many more great factors may persuade your decision to choose a hairstyle that's either an updo, half-up, or all down.

Updos have benefits such as:

- Staying longer longer
- Low maintenance
- Giving your face a lifted look.
- Looking upscale
- Keeps you cooler if you get hot easily
- Having versatility in choosing different styles
- Makes it easy to attach your veil

Because you can't have all positive notions, there are a couple of reasons you should not choose an updo.

Some factors that may dissuade your choice for an updo are the following:

- It will make a round face appear more pronounced
- It can make you look too simplistic if the front of your dress is simple and understated
- It can be heavy and painful to wear if you are not used to having it pinned up
- It may become messy if your hair is resistant to holding its weight

A half-up half-down hairstyle can be thought of as having a timeless appeal. It's a favorite with many modern brides and can work with many different hair lengths and textures. It is a great choice if you like to keep your hair off your face and like practicality. With this hairstyle, you can add twists, braids, bows, or a bouffant.

Similar to the updo, it makes it easy to attach hair accessories, decorative pins, and veils. They can be easily applied as they have a firm structure to be placed into. The bottom portion of the hair can be shown off with waves and curls. The half-up half-down seems to be the best of both worlds.

The comfort level has a lot to do with your choice to wear your hair up or down. Brides that tend to decide to wear their hair all down usually feel most confident and beautiful that way. They are drawn to wearing their hair down on a daily basis. Whether you're thinking about showing off your natural hair texture, enjoy the relaxed look of simplicity. Having your hair all down will look romantic and put your hair on full display.

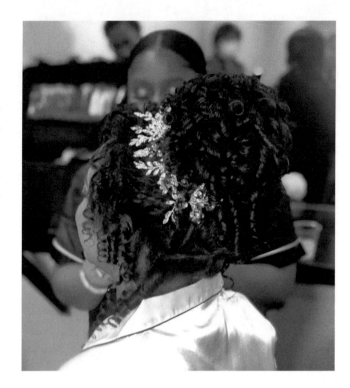

The weather is an important factor to consider when having all of your hair down. Humidity, wind, and rain can play a part in how maintained your hair will stay. Hair that gets frizzy easily will not do well all down if it is styled into a sleek straight finish. Curls will need to be reinforced for long wear with extra hairspray. If there is one thing you can predict, it is Mother Nature. Knowing how your hair normally behaves in the weather conditions and season of the year can help narrow down a style that will perform best under the seasonal conditions surrounding the time of year your wedding is taking place.

There could be a couple of reasons a bride chooses to change her hairstyle for a second look. If your hair is planned to be all down, having a simple backup style in mind will give up options for a second look if your decision doesn't go as planned or if you have an outfit change and want a new hairstyle to match.

Daring brides have opted for a pin curl look styled into an updo or bob to be let out into a curly down style for the reception. Your wedding day is the day to feel like a queen! Why not have queen treatment by having your hairstylist provide a second look?

One thing is certain: you need to choose your hairstyle to flatter your face shape. The different types of shapes vary in wideness, slimness, and roundness, having one pole more prominent than the other and having sharp angles. Choosing a style that works with your unique anatomy is key to defining your beauty and not drawing attention to those areas of your face that make you feel insecure.

Interestingly, the "Oval Rule" can apply to choosing a flattering hairstyle. In the beauty industry, achieving a more oval face shape is the most desirable, proportionate, and balanced. Once you determine your face shape, decisions regarding the best hairstyle will be easier.

Different face shapes include the following:

- Round
- Heart
- Square
- Diamond
- Triangle
- Inverted Triangle
- Rectangle
- Oval

Round

This face shape is very symmetrical in that it has no angles that extend more than the other. The width of the face is the same as the length. You can imagine a perfect circle tracing the face. You want to imagine slimming the sides of the face.

Choosing a hairstyle that has a narrowing effect is most flattering. Having your hair all down can create a linear appearance by minimizing the exposed sides of the face.

Heart

In this face shape, the forehead and cheekbones are a similar width, and the length of the face is longer than the width. You'll want to imagine shortening the face length and narrowing the forehead to give more balance.

Choosing a hairstyle with bangs or a side sweep can create less forehead exposure. If you are uncomfortable with the prominence of your cheekbones, fringed face-framing layers will create more softness.

Square

This shape is similar to a round face but with angles at the side of the jawline and forehead that appear sharp and squared. The length and width of the face are the same, with no pronounced cheekbones. You'll want to lessen the broadness of the forehead and jawline.

Choose a hairstyle that is whimsical and romantic. Lots of curls or waves soften the angular appearance. Face-framing bangs that flow into layers are also a great look.

Diamond

This shape is similar to the heart shape but with a narrowing of the forehead. The widest features are the cheekbones.

Choosing a hairstyle that lessens the peak of the forehead and softens the extension on the cheekbones would be flattering.

Triangle

Starts more narrow at the forehead and gradually gets broader at the jawline, which has a strong angular appearance. More fullness at the top will create a good balance between the prominence of the jawline.

Choosing a hairstyle with a bouffant will be flattering due to it drawing attention and fullness upward. Try some grace-framing curls to soften the angle of the jawline.

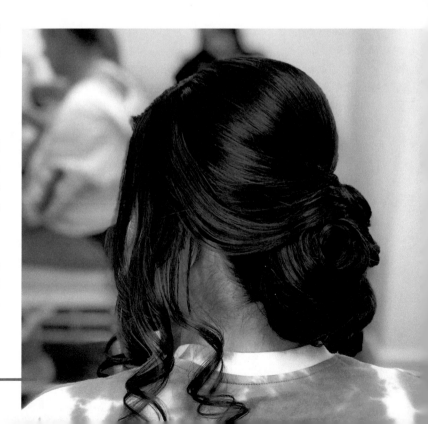

Inverted Triangle

The forehead is the widest measurement, and it gradually gets narrower at the chin. You should avoid layers that get narrow at the end. This gives a more liner illusion and can make the chin look even longer.

Choosing a half-up hairstyle with a center part gives the illusion of a narrower forehead. Face framing pieces that end just above the end of the chin level could visually make it look more balanced. Side-swept bangs or a swoop would be a flattering addition as well. Any hairstyle that covers the wideness of the forehead is best.

Rectangle

Appears to have a long look and is similar to the square. It has strong angles at the side of the jawline and forehead. You should avoid styles that have a blunt cut or finish. The blunt cut mimics the angular look of the face and could make it look emphasized.

Adding texture in the form of soft romantic curls, waves, or layers would be most flattering. The roundness of the texture softens the strong angular appearance. Center-parted long bangs are also a great choice. It should stop before the jawline to have a shortening effect.

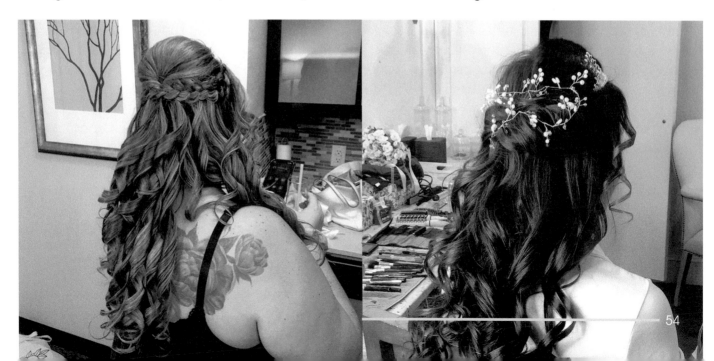

Oval

Since this is the ideal shape, you can pair it with just about any hairstyle. The length of the face is more than the width, and the cheekbones are the most prominent with having the widest appearance.

Now that we've gone over face shapes, you may be wondering which one you have. The best way to determine accurately is by grabbing the measuring tape. Measure the width across your forehead, from ear to ear, and your jawline. Next, take a selfie with your hair pulled back. Research photos of different face shapes and compare them to your own. I also find that asking your mother to assist will give you a clearer picture of the truth. Your mother has studied your face from birth and sometimes can offer the most brutal honesty.

After determining the factors that will be most flattering, you'll be prepared to know what would look the best for your particular features. Gather a few favorite hairstyle inspiration photos and present them to your hairstylist at your bridal trial. You will feel prepared and less indecisive because you've narrowed down specifics that work based on your physical attributes.

Having a hair trial and speaking directly with your artist on the elements of your theme and dress before the big day can ensure you pick the right choice. You'll be relieved to have discussed all your concerns and have your stylist recommend the best plan of action to execute your dream look.

Trials are recommended to be scheduled between 3-6 months before. That should leave plenty of time to reserve your wedding timeframe, have a scheduled timeline of services, and start narrowing down your style preferences. The last thing you'll want to be is panicked and stressed on your wedding day because you're undecided about how to look.

After you've researched and gathered your comfort levels with how you'd like to look, the trial experience should be smooth. You'll feel empowered by having done a personal analysis and feel more confident with the finished product.

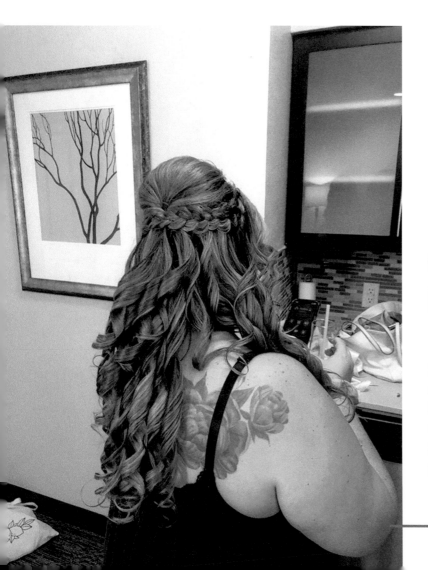

Chapter 8: Hair Extensions

Suppose you've been in awe of all the many celebrities and models in the media having healthy, full long hair and wondered how it was possible. In that case, you're more than likely looking at hair extensions! They come in many different types, colors, and textures.

You can also have flowing goddess hair for your wedding day! Hair extensions are the golden rule for creating a fuller and longer look. In addition, they aid in keeping your look polished. They perform exceptionally well at holding curls longer, sequentially keeping unruly hair looking smoother and preventing fine hair from looking flat after several hours. If you are hesitant to color your hair, extensions can give you a new look by mixing in a different color for a dimensional effect. This is an added benefit for fragile hair or if you like to change up your color often.

Color selection is pretty straightforward. The easiest way to determine color is by choosing the closest to your hair tone. Choosing a lighter tone will be a safe choice if you are deciding between two colors. You can always tone it to a darker shade if it is human hair. In addition, a lighter shade can add a beautiful, dimensional finish.

One major difference between extensions is whether they are bonded in for a semi-permanent effect or a quick temporary addition that can be removed easily without professional assistance. Hair extensions installed by braiding, taping, sewing, gluing, and hot or cold fusion are considered semi-permanent. In contrast, clip-in, ponytails, and flip-in hair are temporary additions.

To make a clear choice between what style extensions to choose, you'll need to consider how long you want them to last, their reusability, how often you use hot tools, and how much time you can devote to maintaining them.

Semi-permanent extensions require the assistance of a salon professional for installation and maintenance. These types should be carefully selected according to your hair type and how often you style your hair regularly. If your hair is fragile, fine, or damaged, it will not be a good solution to add more aggressively bonded techniques. Glued, fusion, and taped hair is great for long wear if caution is used. These methods can last 4-6 months with regular salon maintenance. They have a more involved application and removal process that can damage compromised hair if it is not properly done.

Careful attention must be used while using heat with these methods as well. Heat, heavy conditioners, and oils can cause the fusions to melt, unstick or slip out. If you blow dry and use a flat iron often, you'll minimize the longevity of wear. You should wash and blow dry less frequently. This will expose your hair to less heat to improve its longevity.

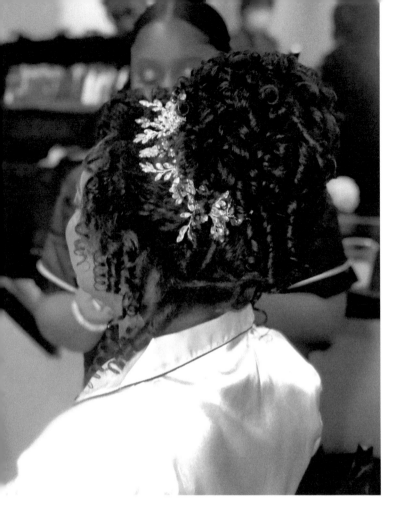

Dry shampoo should become your new bestie, as you'll need to stretch the time between! Washing no more than 1 or 2 times a week will maintain the style and integrity of the extensions. Becoming serious about how you sleep couldn't be more important. Also, using flexible rods and pin curl techniques to preserve any extensions method your hairstyle while sleeping will be best.

A common concern about extensions is whether they will look natural and undetectable. The truth is, having your extensions stand out against your regular has an unpolished, tacky appearance. You should first consider what you'd like the end goal to be over time, then look at texture matching. Since extensions will be an investment, most brides like the idea of reusability.

Look at your lifestyle and regular hair styling routine. More than likely, this will stay consistent. Small changes are to be expected, but if you go out of your way to completely rearrange your styling habits, you may find it daunting. Keep in mind that longer hair will take more time and maintenance. If you are an easy person that doesn't put in time for styling every day, choosing a lower manageable length would be suitable for your lifestyle. Try to use the extensions to create volume and only extend the length a couple more inches than your natural hair. The longer the hair, the more maintenance it will be.

If purchasing clip-in or flip-in hair, the easiest way to go about finding the appropriate length is by measuring. Take a ruler or measuring tape, place it at the base of hair about 2-3 inches up from the bottom of your hairline, then determine how far down you'd like them to fall. This will be the longest point of your hair and how long you should order your extensions. If you want them to be curled, add a couple of inches to your measurements. Curling will lose length. To have them end at the longest point, over-measuring will be appropriate. Typically 20-22 inches works great for updos. It is evident that having too short of hair is limiting for a voluminous chignon or bun.

Your hair texture will play an important role in selection next. Finding extensions close to your natural texture and the final outcome of the design is best. For instance, if your hair is a curly texture and you'd like a smooth bridal hairstyle, choosing a more textured finish, such as wavey or kinky straight, will aid in blending to make it look more seamless when you straighten it. If your hair is curly or coily, choosing a bone-straight texture may run the risk of your hair not matching and standing out from it, especially if the weather turns humid or rainy. If you are having your hair styled into a curly finish and your hair is also curly, curly hair extensions would be perfect.

For blending naturally curly hair with straight extensions, you must ensure your hair is treated to blend properly. Many treatments are great for controlling frizz against humidity and keeping hair more smooth and more controlled. A consultation with your hairstylist will point you in the right direction according to your hair health and tolerability factors. Keep in mind that a permanent treatment will change the inner structure of your hair in the long run. Some semi-permanent treatments that temporarily smooth hair and make it more manageable include a Brazilian blowout, Dominican botox hair treatments, and a keratin treatment.

If you are ready to dive into hair care extensions, be certain that you will spend more time prepping your hair at night, in the morning, and weekly. In addition, if you have them applied semi-permanently, the expense doesn't end with the cost of hair and installation. Regular visits to the salon for deep conditioning, blowouts, and repositioning them is to be expected.

Home care prep will extend the life of your extensions. So you should choose a day or two of the week to follow a routine. The routine should include detangling, washing, deep conditioning and drying.

Things to avoid while wearing extensions are the following:

- Shampooing prior to brushing all tangles out
- Aggressively washing in circles and rubbing
- Sleeping with wet hair
- Letting hair dry without detangling
- Going to bed without putting it in a bun, braid, or scarf

- Leaving in chlorinated or salt water for prolonged periods
- Not using conditioning products
- Using the wrong brush

Doing any of the above will leave severe tangles, dryness, breaking, dullness, and a decreased lifespan.

Many brides love the convenience and ease of clip-in and flip-in hair. If you would like a lower maintenance schedule, like the idea of self-care and fewer salon trips, these methods may be a great fit. They are quick and easy to install, are non-damaging, and can be removed without the assistance of a professional. They should be removed weekly for a wash, detangle and dry session if worn consistently. Hanging them up to dry on a pant hanger makes it extremely easy. They should be dry by the morning.

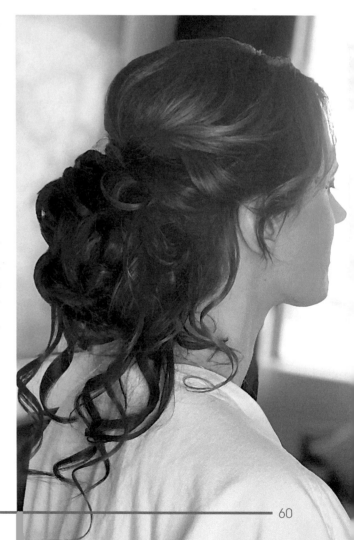

The golden rule to managing hair extensions is to always use a smoothing serum. Apply the serum to the hair while wet to maintain shine and lessen tangles while detangling. Using a straight pin brush versus a brush with ballpoint pins will minimize tearing, breakage, and tangles.

Adding length and volume never sounds like a bad idea, in my opinion! But I do live in Texas. It's practically ingrained in beauty ideals. If you plan to embark on this new journey, make sure you give yourself the appropriate time before your wedding day. Your hair should be in your hands or head at least 3 weeks beforehand. If you plan on using them for a bridal trial, at least 2 months prior would be a sweet spot.

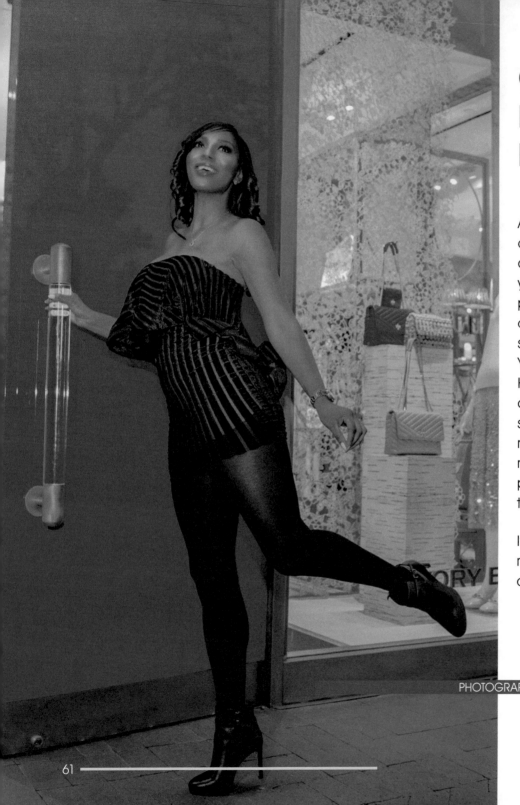

Chapter 9: Hands & Feet Care

Are your hands ready for a close-up? With so much attention put on showing off your pretty ring and shoes, putting grooming attention on your hands and feet should be on the schedule. Yes, you read that right! Having it scheduled on your calendar can prevent it from slipping your mind. With so many other requirements needing your attention in the planning process, it can be the last thing to remember.

If you don't already have regular appointments for a manicure and pedicure,

PHOTOGRAPHER MAJID IRAVANI

now is the time to splurge. Not only should you keep up the maintenance schedule, but it is equally important to have a moment to destress and relax. It can be like a piece of heaven to break away from the many duties of planning. Some brides also invite their bridesmaids and mothers to enjoy a special pampering day leading up to their wedding. To have your nails, hands, and feet looking fresh and polished, you should plan on a spa visit the week of your wedding.

In the time leading up to the wedding, you also should set aside time for self-maintenance. Investigate what concerns you most about your feet and hands so that you may create a plan to combat your concerns. A few popular complaints include excessive dryness, sweating, nail-biting, callousness, dark knuckles, fragile peeling nails, and hyperpigmentation from scars.

A remedy to help combat hand dryness and hyperpigmentation is a mask with honey, collagen, or vitamin E. The mask must be done apart from a weekly schedule for the best benefits. Although many of these types of masks can be purchased at your local beauty store or online, making them yourself can be a cost-effective and fun solution!

Recipe for a honey mask:

- 2 tbsp of honey
- 1/4 cup of sugar
- 1/3 cup of olive oil
- Steamed towel

Directions: mix all ingredients. Then smooth the mixture over your hands while rubbing them together for a few minutes. Put your hands on disposable gloves, then wrap them in a warm steamed towel until it cools. Take off the gloves, rinse off your hands, pat dry, and add your favorite hand cream.

Both honey and Vitamin E oil have a long history of treating and healing dryness. It has antioxidant and anti-aging properties. With consistent use, it can diminish fine lines and wrinkles and lighten hyperpigmentation from scars.

To keep the softening effects of your treatments, apply your favorite hand and foot cream and seal with an oil or petroleum jelly. If you are brave enough, sleeping with your hands in moisturizing cotton gloves after your treatment intensifies the results.

Fiona Taylor

Hand and feet sweating can be both embarrassing and uncomfortable. If you throw nerves in the mix, what was once something of a small concern can become a large dilemma. Sweaty feet can make your Cinderella moment too storybook-perfect when losing a shoe during your walk down the aisle or a staircase was not a part of the plan!

Thankfully, these are remedies for controlling excessive perspiration:

- Baking soda- this magical ingredient mixed with water left on for 5 minutes or thereabout and then rinsed can act as a long-acting antiperspirant.
- Apple cider vinegar- apply this daily for detoxing effects
- Talcum powder- Apply before you put on your shoes. It will keep absorbing moisture and control odor.

Next to foot appearance is foot health. As a bride, I'm sure you are all too familiar with foot pain from wearing heels! Because cute shoes are not always the most comfortable, you'll find it a very good idea to plan ahead to minimize discomfort.

Adding a healthy foot routine is essential to more than just looking great for your wedding day. If you continue taking care of your feet, it can be worthwhile in the long run. Foot stretching has many benefits that prepare you for long hours of standing and dancing. It can also come in handy for providing additional support for long meetings,

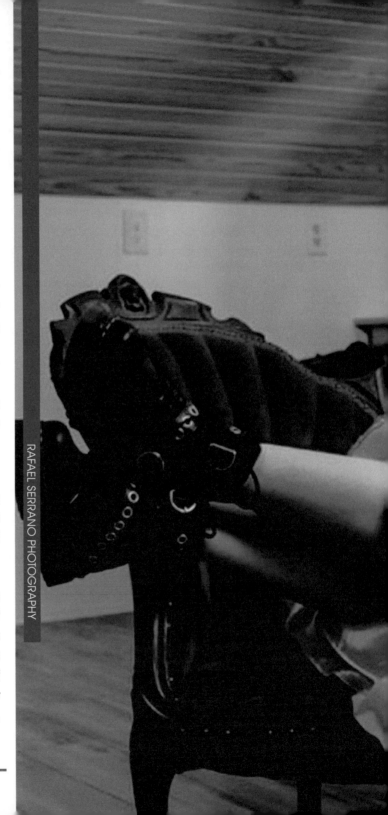

RAFAEL SERRANO PHOTOGRAPHY

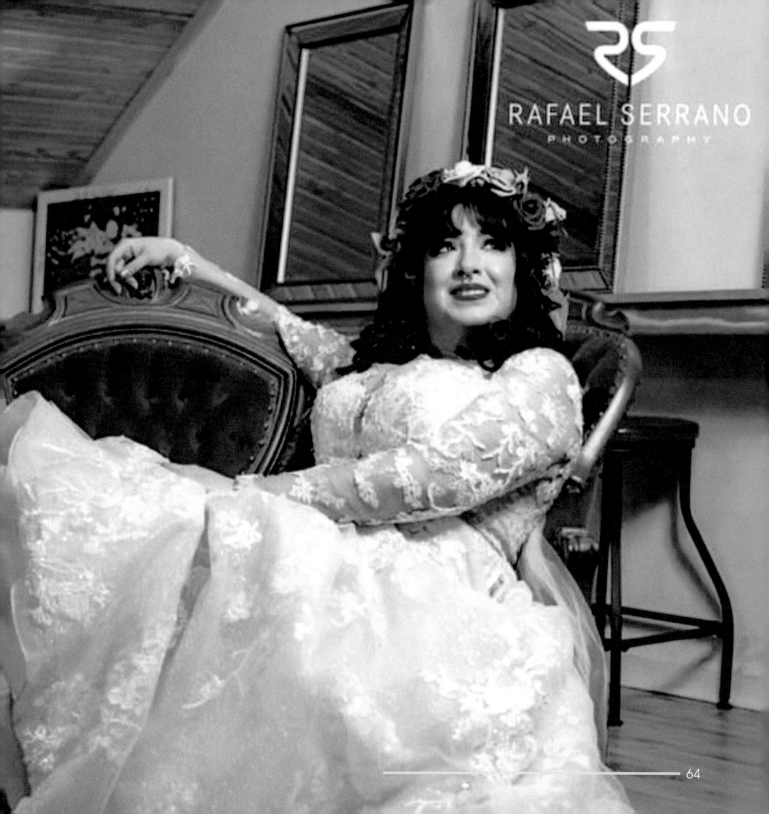

RS
RAFAEL SERRANO
PHOTOGRAPHY

64

attending other events, conferences, prior to working out, or otherwise any future times you'll need to have your feet be cooperative.

The benefits of stretching include improving flexibility and range of motion, alleviating pain, and improving circulation. It also helps keep the feet and ankles strong, which helps reduce the chances of a sprained ankle. Since your feet have a lot to do with your posture, you may find that keeping them flexible and strong will keep other joints properly aligned and prevent joint and back pain.

If you've found yourself running into a chair, person, or wall regularly, chances are you could use balance improvement. Stretching your feet will strengthen your foot muscles to hold up your body, so it is not flying into objects mistakenly. Walking gracefully is certainly a skill that will help you when you are wearing a heavy gown. In addition to the weight of your gown, nerves could make you feel dizzy. This goes without saying, but not many people consider how drinking champagne and alcoholic drinks will affect your balance. As you see, there are a lot of factors that coincide with having a great balance for your wedding day. Stretching may assist in preparation for both unexpected surprises and expected partying.

In addition to helping your feet have an improved range of motion, strengthening them will put emphasis on improving endurance. A very good way to do that is by strengthening the muscles in your feet. First, identify what areas cause you discomfort while standing for prolonged periods. Putting more focus on building strength and flexibility in those areas will help isolate what in particular you can benefit from.

Below are some exercises with directions that target your foot and ankle muscles:

- Toe curls with a towel- While barefooted, sit down in a chair. Place a towel on the floor in front of you. Find a lightweight object such as a book or paperweight and place it at the opposite end. Scrunch your toes by gathering up the towel to bring it toward you. Do about 15 repetitions.
- Heel and toe raise- While sitting or standing, simply raise your heel off the ground about 15 times. Next, rock your foot back onto your heel and raise your toes off the ground 15 times
- Short foot- While sitting in a chair, put both feet on the ground. Keep your heels and toes touching the floor, and lift your arch up. Hold for a few seconds and relax. Repeat 15 times.
- Balancing- Stand up and lift one leg off the ground. Hold this position for 15 seconds, then switch legs. For varying degrees of difficulty, try lowering your leg to the floor and raising it back up slowly while trying to maintain balance. Repeat 15 times.

The sooner you start improving your foot strength and balance, the better. Not only will your feet benefit from these exercises, but your legs will also tone up, which isn't a bad idea for showing off on your honeymoon!

Taking time to choose the correct size shoe is one of the most important aspects of the actual shoe design. Continually wearing the wrong size shoe can contribute to health challenges, unsightly blisters, corns, deformations, and unwarranted pain. Hence, thinking of ways to welcome comfort in all areas of your wardrobe should be at the front of your mind.

The perfect shoe size should be identified by many factors. Knowing what size you normally wear is a great start, but realizing that shoe manufacturers vary slightly should be considered. One size 8 in one company could be 7.5 or 8.5 in another. Unbeknown to most, one foot is slightly larger than the other. Consider taking your measurements from your larger foot for the most accurate result.

When shoe shopping, decide on a time in the late afternoon or evening. This is an ideal time because

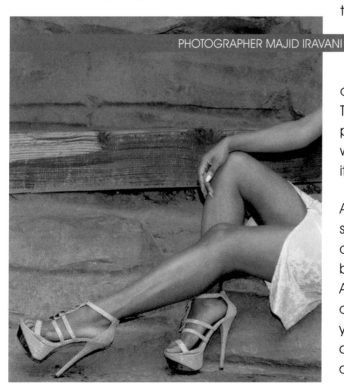

PHOTOGRAPHER MAJID IRAVANI

the feet will have swelled a bit and resemble what you may encounter from being on your feet all day. Both feet should be measured to determine which of the two is the larger one. Having a bit of toe wiggle is to be expected. The toes should never feel crammed in, and the pinky toe should not feel pinched. If it's been a while since your last shoe fitting, you should make it a priority when shopping for your wedding day.

Adding inserts to the inside of your shoes can save you a great deal of pain. The most useful areas to cushion include the ball of your feet, the back of your heels, and the joints of your toes. Adding a heel cushion to the back of your shoes can not only prevent an unexpected slip out of your shoe. But it can be a lifesaver for preventing a painful blister from the amount of walking and dancing around you will be doing. If your feet will be enclosed, it won't hurt to wrap a couple of toes in moleskin tape.

Lastly, the worst pain of all: the ball of your foot! I would suggest doubling your cushion with one inside the shoes and adding a rubber no-skid shoe grip on the bottom. These easy tricks are just what grandma ordered! Although you may have feet dressed like your grandmother, don't let that dissuade you from having comfortable feet. The last thing you want is to focus on your aching feet while trying to pose pretty for pictures.

When all else fails, and you still have foot pain, bring the necessities to numb the sensation. While this is only a temporary fix, all you have to do is spray down your feet with a lidocaine foot spray and pop a pain reliever. You just need to get to the end of the night. If you made it to the end of the night with numb feet, welcome to the glamour club!

As the old saying goes, you get what you pay for. Quality shoes should be an investment. Not only should they look amazing, but they should also be functional. New shoes should feel comfortable from the first day you purchase them. Breaking in shoes is something to be expected, but only to allow the shoe to form your unique foot structure. You should avoid shoes that feel painful to stand in or walk across a short distance. A test of how they feel on hard floors and carpets should be done.

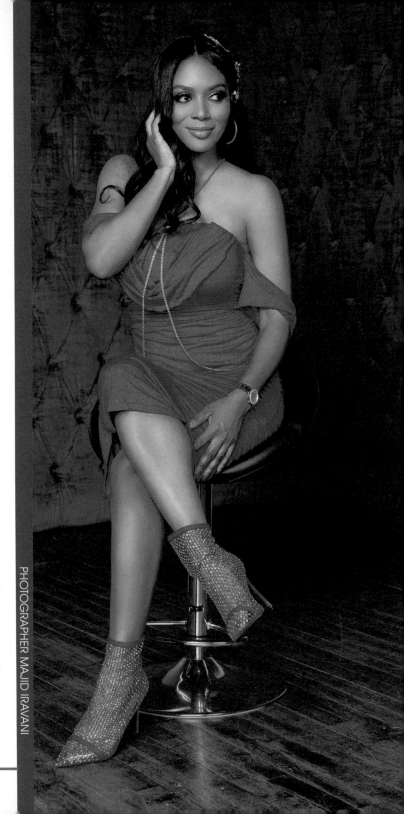

PHOTOGRAPHER MAJID IRAVANI

Getting your shoes ready for a long exposure is a task that should not go unchecked. After my years working in proximity to shoe departments while employed as a counter makeup artist, one piece of advice that really stuck with me was that you should wear your new shoes around the house at night. Wearing them while doing chores to loosen stiffness up and have them mold to your foot is ingenious. It's also a fast solution to getting your feet acclimated to walking easily in heels. One thing is for sure: shoes that are either too small or too big can affect how graceful you appear. You don't want your feet flopping around and out of your shoes. You also do not want to be tip-toeing around, curled over in pain. I can attest one of the worst pains you could feel is in your feet!

Doing chores in heels doesn't just make you look ultra glamorous but allows the material to give way to what's to come. Another way to prepare them is by manually massaging them from the interior. The shoe stretcher tool is also useful in relaxing tight toes in narrow closed-toe toes. Preparing your shoes for wear doesn't just end there. Chances are you'll be walking from different locations for your bridals and first-look photos. The outside elements can stain the fabric. If you are not open to dying them another color after your big day, sealing them with a waterproof protectant will come in handy for blocking stains. Mud or dirt on white satin heels is nearly impossible to remove.

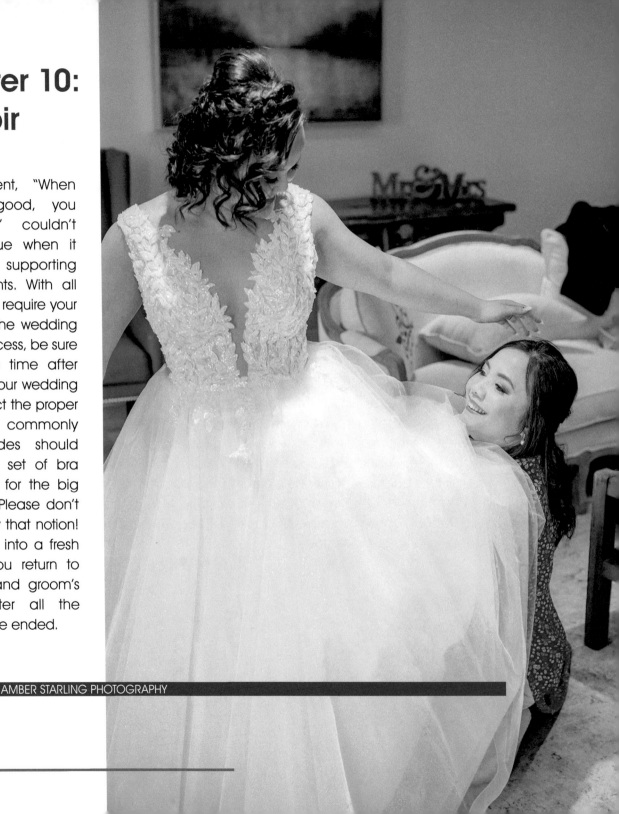

Chapter 10: Boudoir

The statement, "When you look good, you feel good," couldn't be more true when it comes to supporting undergarments. With all the tasks that require your attention in the wedding planning process, be sure to set aside time after purchasing your wedding dress to select the proper lingerie. It's commonly thought brides should have a frilly set of bra and panties for the big reveal later. Please don't be fooled by that notion! You can slip into a fresh set when you return to your bride and groom's quarters after all the festivities have ended.

AMBER STARLING PHOTOGRAPHY

Since you'll be on display for all to see, you should be certain you make your undergarment purchase in accordance with how to flatter your figure in your dress design. Far too many brides arrive with the wrong type of bra or flashy colored panties that affects their final appearance. You should keep in mind that photos will capture every angle. Bra straps, bands, raised textures, and the color of your undergarments should be concealed properly for a classy finish.

The first step to identifying which undergarments to choose is by looking at your dress cut details. After you've purchased your dream dress, take photos of how you look in it from all angles. Take note of the neckline in the front and the back, the tightness, the sheerness, how the fabric lays, what type of fabric it is, and the skirt design. Paying close attention to what can make your dress look more flattering on your figure and give you a confidence boost is key. Using your first dress fitting can prove worthwhile in allowing you to see exactly where changes can be made to enhance your figure. Having your mother come along while dress shopping or a brutally honest close friend can assist with identifying what modifications can be done to support and can enhance your appearance. Investigate what bulges are noticed that can be smoother and what can be lifted, synched, or puffed up. This will give clarity into setting the direction of the necessary undergarments and make up look like a million-dollar bride!

Different types of shapewear can assist with defining your figure and eliminate bloatedness and bulges. First and foremost, you should keep your comfort in mind. Buying shapewear that is either too small or a low-quality grade is incredibly uncomfortable. It can add more problems than it solves, such as rolling down, riding up, painfully poking, pinching, or constricting your breathing. Depending on your dress design, top choices include bodysuits, tummy control thongs, shaping shorts, high-waisted skirts, and shaping briefs, to name a few.

Shapewear comes in varying compression levels and may contain boning or built-in bras. If you're looking for more contouring, selecting a style with boning and a higher compression will give you more shaping. If you desire a little support but care more about a relaxed and comfortable feeling, high-waisted briefs offer more flexibility with added support. Wearing your selected shapewear a time or two before your big day is ideal. This will break it in a little and provide first-hand experience of whether you can last hours wearing it.

When getting your dress altered, depending on the style of the bodice, you could potentially have a bra sewn in good added support. Choosing to go braless is a personal choice, and you should be familiar with the feeling and choice before the actual day. There are times and factors when going braless diminishes the classiness of your appearance. There are plenty of fashion tricks to keep your breasts supported and appear like you're not wearing a bra. Some to name include stick-on bras, boob tape, and pasties. These can offer freedom and a no-hassle experience. There's no worse feeling than your strapless bra slipping down and needing to readjust it in its rightful place. It feels dreadful, and the adjusting process looks unclassy.

If you're a no-fuss type of bride and don't like the idea of constricting shapewear, you may like the idea of wearing tights. I personally love the effect of pantyhose and tights. They are great for covering blemishes on your legs and smoothing your figure. You can skip shaving and can even go commando! Depending on the season, you may find that they provide functionality in keeping you warm in the colder months and dry in the heat. They are wonderful for preventing chafing and can prove beneficial in preventing blisters on your feet. Although pantyhose and tights have many positive attributes, I'm sure you are all too familiar with how uncomfortable they can feel when you wear a pair of lower quality. You simply don't want to skimp on quality for such an important occasion and find yourself itching and scratching down the aisle.

Not only does wearing the proper supporting undergarments prove vital to enhancing your figure and comfort, but it can also be important for the structure of the dress design. Slips are great for giving your gown added shaping and functionality when walking. A common insecurity among brides is that everyone will watch as they walk down the aisle. In fact, everyone will be watching the bride everywhere she goes. It is a good idea to walk around and move in ways you are naturally inclined to move to see how the dress behaves and if the fabric wraps around your feet and slips between your legs. The right slip can assist in bowing out the hem of your gown to allow you to walk more seamlessly. While not every dress needs a slip, you can certainly benefit from them if you find that your legs become entangled in the fabric maneuvering around. Think about dancing as well.

Generally, gowns are made without additional fluffing under the skirt to allow the bride to modify the fullness level according to her preferences. While wearing your wedding gown at one of your fittings, determine how full you would like the skirt to be. The underskirts are available in two distinct styles. For example, a hoop slip that has boning that wraps around the skirt to bow it out and a full crinoline slip that has layers of tulle to create fullness.

Your seamstress can assist in taking the proper measurements needed for ordering and suggest which slip will give the best look for your gown design.

By searching more into the designer of the gown and the dress design specifications, you can find more information on the proper terminology for your skirt style. The dress or alterations shop may also provide you with this information. Below are the types of petticoat slip styles for reference:

- A line
- Two hoop
- Three hoop
- Six hoop
- Train
- Mermaid

By this point, you may be wondering how you'll be able to use the bathroom wearing all these undergarments. Having a plan in place before the occurrence will save you worry and ease your mind. A close friend or mother may need to assist you. Purchasing a bridal bathroom helping slip is

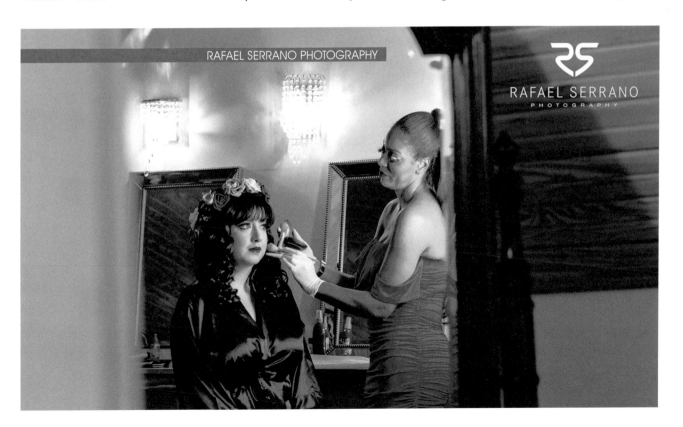
RAFAEL SERRANO PHOTOGRAPHY

RAFAEL SERRANO
PHOTOGRAPHY

Fiona Taylor

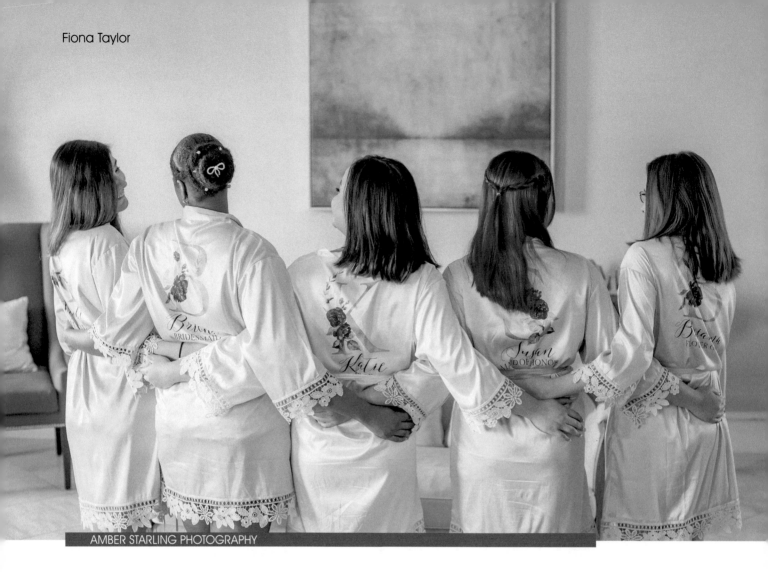

AMBER STARLING PHOTOGRAPHY

also an option if you desire privacy. A couple of great inventions take the guesswork out of using the restroom in a full gown.

One thing that brides tend to underestimate is the amount of time they will spend prepping. It's important to understand that beauty takes time. If you've ever tried to rush getting ready, you are more than likely to experience heightened nerves, disheveled clothing, messily applied cosmetics, and less-than-desirable hair styling. Cutting time off here may affect how you show up for the entirety of

73

your event. Since you'll be spending ample time getting ready, ensure you dress to your comfort and for great photos.

Planning how everyone looks while getting ready may seem over the top now, but you must keep in mind that you will be photographed and filmed the entire day. Showing up in your baggy T-shirt and sweats may seem comfortable but will not show you in the best light. It's also worthwhile to imagine how easily you can change out of your outfit. Tight collars that pull over your head are not ideal due to the likelihood of them fraying your hairstyle and smearing your makeup. A garment that opens easily from the front is suggested. Choosing a beautiful button-down shirt and shorts set or a glamorous robe will allow for dressing functionality and look great in photos. It's your day to shine, and it's your living documentary. Looking good from all angles should be at the front of your mind!

When you plan your boudoir wardrobe, it should incorporate your theme for cohesiveness. While you do not need to pick every color in your palette, choosing your main theme elements and color will pair perfectly. It's a popular choice to have all the bridesmaids in matching robes and you in a fancier version or white. Not only is it a good idea that everyone matches, but robes also make great gifts for your bridesmaids and mothers.

The theme of your wedding should play a part in the type of garments you choose for getting ready. Think of the venue and vibes of your decoration. Is

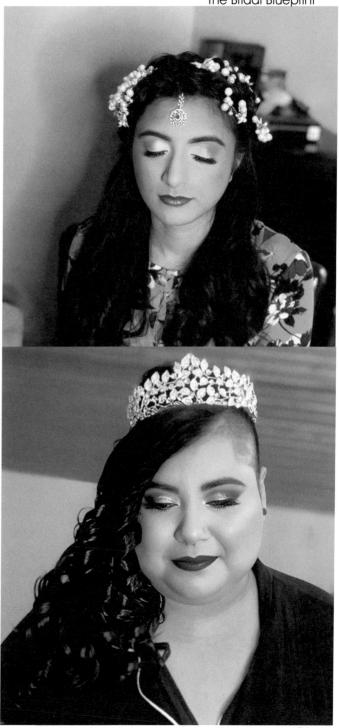

it upscale, boho chic, western, modern, fun, relaxed, or retro? Using your theme as a keyword in your search can assist in narrowing down the complimenting garment options.

It's one thing to look cute in your boudoir clothes but another to ensure you stay fresh. As mentioned prior, please do not wear your frilly bedroom lingerie under your wedding dress. You'll feel much more comfortable in undergarments that allow you to look great in your wedding dress while offering support. Typically, cute lingerie is designed to look cute but is not always the most comfortable to wear for prolonged periods. Since you will be close to people assisting you to get dressed and even use the bathroom, managing hygiene is important.

Baby/feminine hygiene wipes are excellent to have on hand for refreshing your body, underarms, and groin areas. They are a perfect complement to the bathroom. Also, they can be a valuable resource to keep you shower-fresh while you're running around managing wedding day duties. Often, you may find yourself traveling between different photoshoot locations in hot environments. Nerves also play a part in sweating more than normal. Having a cool wipe-down is the perfect refresher.

As mentioned in a prior chapter, dusting powder will keep your feet from becoming odorous and sweaty and is also a good idea for other bodily areas prone to perspiration. Dusting it on your panties, back, and in areas that fold and frequently rub back and forth will keep you dry and clean. If dusting powder is not your style, the intimate deodorant spray is another great product. It is mess free and has an easy application in hard-to-reach areas.

Depending on how open your friends and family members are regarding bodily functions, chances are you may have heard someone say their menstruation cycle started on their big day. Although tracking your period is a great idea to prevent any surprising debuts of Aunt Flow, it isn't always reliable. As someone who works with brides on a weekly basis, I can attest to its truth! It totally happens. Many women find that taking birth control lessens the risk.

Planning and executing an event so large as your wedding day is extremely stressful and straining on the body. Stress in high amounts is known to affect the hypothalamus part of the brain that controls hormones. This, in turn, can kick-start a women's cycle early and make it arrive sooner than expected. As unfortunate as it may sound, planning for the unexpected is the best plan. It may not be you that could have a surprise monthly visit, but it could be anyone else in your bridal party. Bring back-up feminine supplies and inform your bridal party just in case anyone needs them.

Chapter 11: Grace & Beauty Etiquette

You've made it! Your dream of becoming the most charming bride is at your fingertips. Before we can celebrate, I must remind you that you are only as beautiful as you act. Letting your actions lead more than your beauty can serve as a great pearl of wisdom. Keeping your mannerisms and beauty classy can make you appear even more stunning. There's nothing more unbefitting than a beautiful person with an ugly attitude and unrefined social behavior.

One certain thing is we've all heard the endless bridezilla stories from family and friends. While this may be one of the biggest moments of your life, it is quintessential for your sanity and health that you remain in control of your emotions. One way to remain calm and overcome a meltdown is by taking time with the planning process. Often, the reasons for explosions of anger come from anxiety from not being in control or being unprepared.

Indecision is the enemy of success. Hence, taking time to dissect the elements of your theme and personal style can help make decisions clearer.

Think about how organized you are naturally. If you feel overwhelmed, it's time to delegate some of the tasks to either a professional planner or coordinator or a willing bridal party participant skilled in the organization area.

Hiring skilled professionals to assist in making sure everything runs smoothly and looks cohesive will allow you to remain on schedule and have peace of mind. On average, the typical time for planning a wedding is six months to one year. One common mistake is to wait until a couple of months before reserving vendors. Indeed, starting right away with research and development is best. This way, the chances of getting your dream vendors are more likely. Professional vendors generally require a contract and a retainer to secure your time frame. Remember that you are hiring the most elite professionals for special

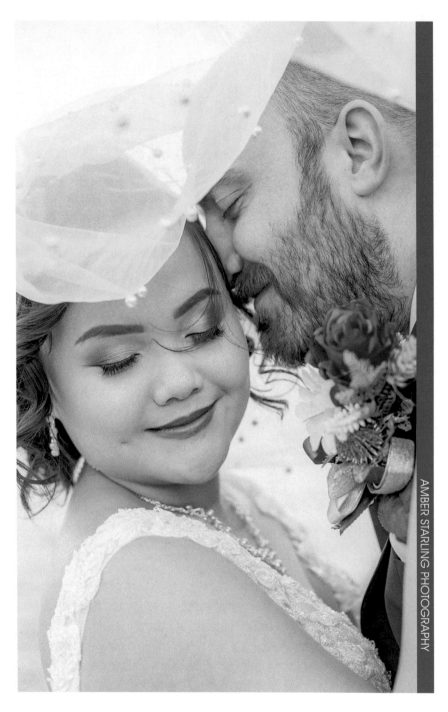

AMBER STARLING PHOTOGRAPHY

events. A vendor specializing in weddings is in one of the most elite event categories! More than likely, one that comes with more experience and a higher price tag to ensure your special day is flawless. Many companies are willing to offer payment plans if you inquire!

When you have made a choice to hire a professional, chances are they specialize in the trade they offer. They can give you a clear idea of what to expect based on their industry experience. Listening to their suggestions and recommendations come from prior experiences with past bridal bookings. Using discretion while speaking can show good manners and courteousness. Allowing others to speak and completely convey their intended suggestions will give you a well-rounded point of view and be less confrontational.

If this is your first go around, try to remain flexible in what advice is given to you for the best results and outcome. With this said, be sure to do your research and comparison to find the best suitable vendor that aligns with your end goal. This is one sure way to prevent a disaster before it happens.

This is your day to look the most beautiful that you will ever look in your life. Even if it's just for a couple hours or one day, your photos and memories will last a lifetime. They will be framed to hang on your wall for all to see. Wedding photos are often shared from one generation to the next. Since many brides are newcomers to many aspects of planning for a big event, it is worthwhile to experience a preview or bridal trial. Testing, feeling, seeing, and even tasting can be fun parts of the planning experience!

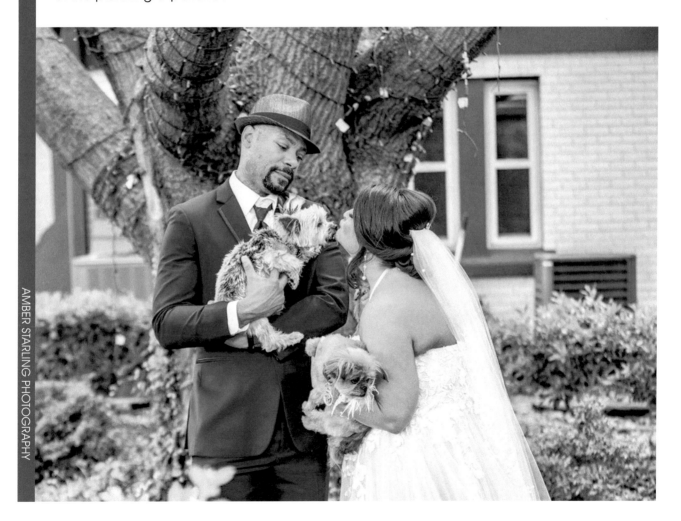

AMBER STARLING PHOTOGRAPHY

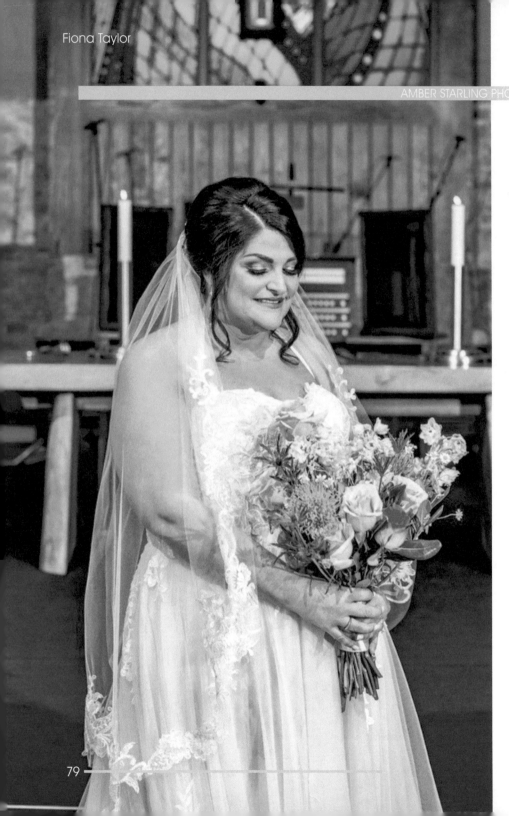

AMBER STARLING PHOTOGRAPHY

Because so much pressure is put on looking absolutely fabulous, setting up a bridal trial will ease some nerves and allow you to have a sneak peek into what you'll experience on the wedding day. Nerves and anxiety can make you feel indecisive. If you've never had professional-grade beauty services before, you most certainly should not forgo a trial. Makeup and hair done specifically for photography differ from what you may be used to. Beauty has the power to shift emotions to make you feel empowered, more confident, and shine. On the other hand, it can also be overwhelming and prompt feelings of insecurity if you are unfamiliar with it. Trying it out to gather your comfort level is the best way to decide what can make you feel and look beautiful.

Regarding beauty services, certain behaviors can assist in making the process go smoothly and ensure you are respectful to the service provider. Before your makeup and hair process starts, your beauty professional should thoroughly understand your comfort levels, theme, and wedding colors. It is essential to choose inspirational photos of makeup and hairstyles that speak to you. Since makeup preferences are unique to each person, a photo will give the artist a good starting place to understand your tastes.

During services, you should be an open book and listen to the suggestions of how makeup and hair can be styled to best define your features. Makeup for photographs should be applied with a heavier hand for it to photograph properly to avoid looking washed out and applied adequately to cover imperfections that otherwise peek through the magnification level of HD photo and video equipment. Sometimes this may be a different technique from what you're used to. There are slight differences in how a person looks in photos versus in real life.

If there are any hard dislikes or allergies to any products, be sure to make those known so that they will not get applied. Although it may be tough not to look in the mirror at the process, it is common courtesy not to watch the entire process unless you receive a one-on-one lesson. There are appropriate times when looking at the progress is required, and you'll be prompted to include feedback. It's a good idea to speak up and mention appropriate feedback at those times so modifications can be easily made.

During beauty services, hygiene attention is strongly encouraged. Ensure that your face is a clean canvas free of makeup and that your teeth are brushed prior. Also, during services, avoid smoking, vaping, sneezing, or coughing without covering your mouth. Importantly, avoid eating until after the service is completed. It may seem like common territory, but it may not be a thought if you are completely new to receiving beauty services. Behaviors normally associated with your home comforts must be modified in a professional setting. Also, products used by beauty professionals need to stay at a pristine level of hygiene because they are used on multiple people.

Learning how to carry yourself elegantly is a task to be handled. You must now think of yourself as royalty awaiting your big debut. This is exactly how you will look and how people will treat you. You must also act the part. You should live up to every moment that you're center stage. With this said, there are certain behaviors that you can exhibit to make you look more elegant.

How you walk and carry yourself allows you to stand out as the most beautiful and dreamy person in the room. Careful attention must be paid to the finishing touches of your clothing and posture. All wrinkles should be steamed out of your veil and gown, as well as unmatching jewelry and hair bands removed from your wrists.

If you've followed prior instructions in choosing the correct undergarments, you'll be in a good starting place. Constantly tugging at a slipping bra, rolling panty lines, or poking boning should be avoided. It is not classy to constantly be consumed with adjusting your clothing or, worse, undergarments.

It may feel strange at first, but practicing being hyper-aware of your mannerisms can be extremely helpful in allowing you to look more graceful. Notice how often you touch your hair, scratch your head, scratch your face, adjust your clothes, run into furniture, slouch while sitting, lean while standing, and lose your balance or footing. Focus on adjusting those less-than-flattering mannerisms so you can show up great from every angle.

When you walk, slow down your pace a smidge. Practice taking small steps to maintain control and range. Some gown styles, such as a mermaid, limit your gait. In addition, if your slip is a hoop style, fast walking may rock the skirt like a bell back and forth. The idea is to make it seem like you are simply gliding effortlessly across the floor.

Since you may be walking in different terrains throughout the day, practice walking gracefully, similar to your bridal shoes on carpet, grass, wooden floors, and even on unlevel gravel if you plan a country-style ceremony. In most cases, keeping your feet balanced and steady on the balls of your feet can help avoid sinking stilettos in the grass and wobbling on gravel. Building up your calf muscles will be a worthwhile venture.

Getting used to walking in a long gown can be made easy by remembering to prepare your step. Grabbing the sides of the skirt and then lifting it off the ground to expose the front of your shoes will assist if you are walking up or down straits and on uneven ground. If your dress is hemmed longer than you're used to, walking while slightly kicking your feet up with each step will eliminate tripping on the front of the dress. Also, the trick of holding one side up a bit is functional and very classy while dancing.

It is pretty standard to have your dress bustled during alterations and fittings for easy walking during your reception. If your train is short, bustling may not be necessary. In these cases, learning to walk around is vital. If you imagine a person standing directly behind you, you would obviously not turn around sharply

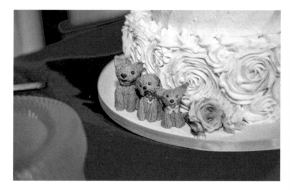
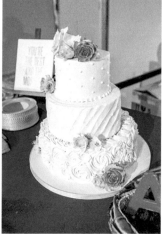
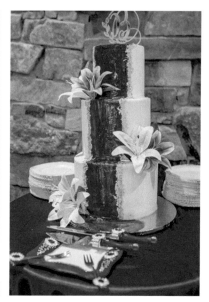

AMBER STARLING PHOTOGRAPHY

and walk straight into them. It is a similar situation with a train. Start by turning to either side and walk around in a circular movement to avoid stepping on the train.

When it comes to sitting down in your dress, it is easier to manage than walking around in it. Gathering the bulk of the fluff and shifting it to the front before you sit will avoid any strange feelings of fabric pulling. If your dress is a silky material, making sure the back is flat against the chair will lessen the chances of the back becoming wrinkled. When in doubt, sit in the chair using your hip first, then shift slowly over to having your back aligned straight. This works perfectly for ball gowns with hoop slips.

Now that you're sitting properly, you are ready for table manners. Proper table manners are a sign of refinement. One of my favorite pieces of advice for brides is, "Eat and drink pretty!" However, this advice is mostly given to help keep your lipstick from wearing off prematurely. Having your lipstick worn for 4-6 hours is possible, even through eating and drinking. Here are some tricks and tips that are worthwhile to practice for flawless execution:

- Try to eat small bites.
- Do not let your utensils constantly rub against your lips.
- Place food directly and carefully into your mouth.
- Use your teeth to slide off the food while it's in your slightly closed mouth.

- Eat more slowly.
- Drink from the same place on a cup.

Following these techniques will not only keep your mouth from becoming messy but also assist you in eating more ladylike. Some other important subjects to mention are basic table manners. Your napkin should be the first thing you touch when you sit down. Ladies always drape the napkin across their lap and fold it in half, with the opening of the fold facing their bodies. When the napkin is used, it should be dabbed using one side and placed on the corners of your mouth gently to absorb food and moisture, leaving your lipstick intact. Som e lipstick transfer is completely ok. When finished, it is then placed back on the lap with the messy side within the fold.

When chewing your food, keep your mouth closed and avoid making loud noises. Take your time eating by choosing small bites so that you can leave moments for easy conversation. Also, try to avoid speaking with food in your mouth. If, for any reason, you should need to answer a question right away, covering your mouth with your hand while speaking is a polite gesture. Food particles flying out of your mouth is not a good look.

If you are not used to formal dining etiquette, you should frequently practice at home. Incorporate good manners around your family and friends in an informal and formal setting. If you are an overachiever, practicing dining etiquette by yourself is the way to go!

A good rule of thumb is to not slouch and be too relaxed at the dinner table. Sitting upright with your back against the chair is a proper position. This naturally will limit the urge to place your elbows on the table. Also, your forearms should be the only body part on the table. The idea is to always maintain a formal appearance.

If you've heard the expression in movies where ladies mention they need to powder their noses after dinner, you can conclude that they have good table manners. At the end of eating, you may be tempted to touch up your makeup right away at the dinner table. But it should be mentioned that any makeup application that requires a mirror should be done in the ladies' room. Lip gloss and lip balm can pass so long as you're not looking into a mirror.

Your trip to the restroom may also include other touch-up duties such as hand washing, brushing your hair, using a toothpick, and refreshing makeup.

Conclusion

Remember our bride from the beginning? She had the most fantastic wedding of her dreams! I was there before she arrived and assisted her into the hours of her reception to ensure she remained immaculate for dancing, partying, and pictures. Surprisingly to us both, her body's reaction to hyperhidrosis was caused by a mixture of the weight of her wedding gown, nerves, and Texas heat.

Unfortunately, some situations can occur that you simply can not foresee until they happen. Nonetheless, a spontaneous burst of perspiration is now on the list! After coming in contact with countless brides, I was made aware that they were, in one way or another, caught in moments where emergency assistance was required. I, in return, learned invaluable information and tools of the trade to professionally assist them.

I hope to equip ladies with information to empower them through education and preparedness. My goal is to lessen the circumstances that could potentially be catastrophic and disappointing for a bride.

I felt called to write this book because I saw a need for a comprehensive analysis that could assist brides in making sure they know what factors go into helping them look their best for one of the most important days of their lives.

Preparing to be dreamy for your wedding day comes with preparation and planning. However, not doing research and self-discovery can have dire consequences. Deciding to look beautiful is only half of the work. The other half is dissecting what that means to you so you don't end up wearing an unsuitable look.

This guide will help you navigate the factors crucial for the longevity of your look, help determine your personal tastes, how to correlate your look properly with your wedding theme, and be perceived as the most charming lady in the room with etiquette training.

You've now obtained industry secrets and an in-depth knowledge of the processes involved in a beauty transformation. So you should feel empowered in making the right choices to become the most dreamy version of yourself! Using this valuable information will prove worthwhile in developing a solid beauty plan as well as suitably aligned discussions with your hired beauty professionals who can assist in making your dream look come to fruition.

Fiona Taylor

To learn more about other bridal success stories and view my company's professional bridal service offerings, please visit www.facesbyfiona.com.

Congratulations, and welcome to the new you!

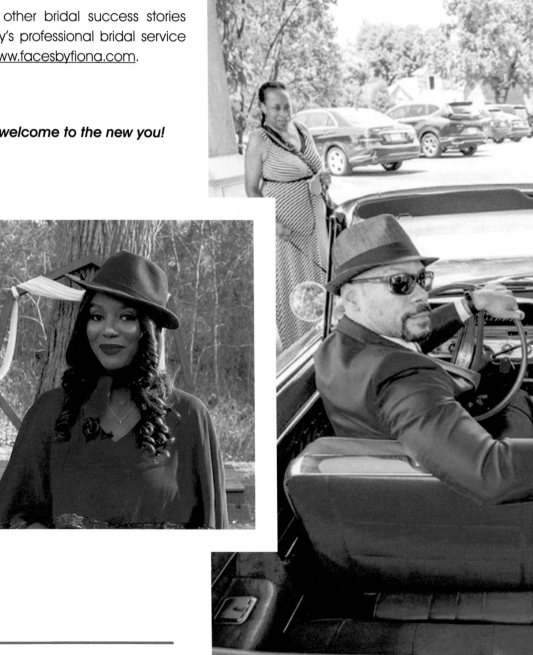

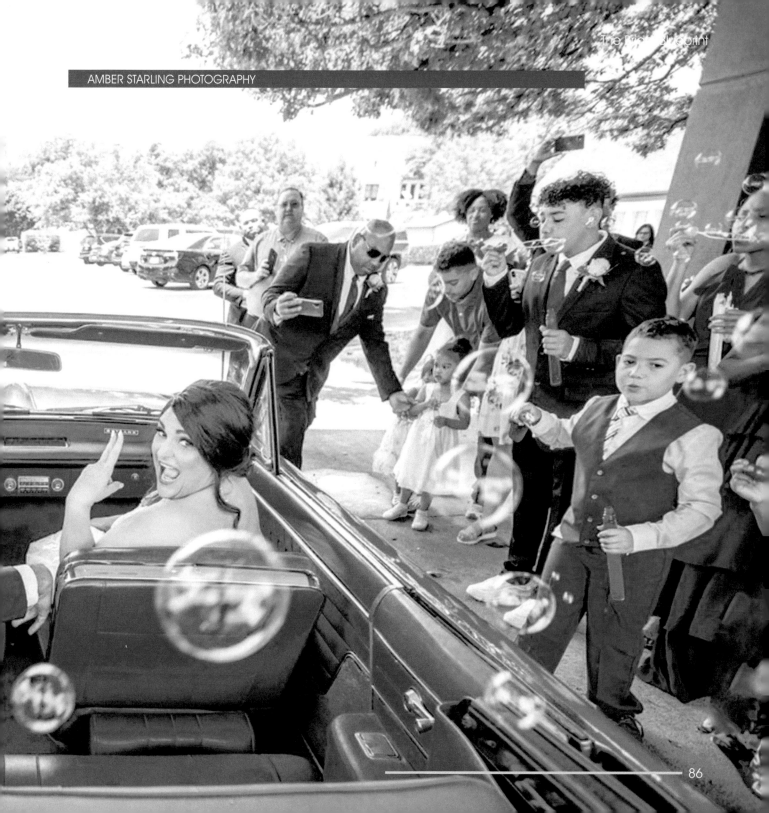

AMBER STARLING PHOTOGRAPHY

Printed in the United States
by Baker & Taylor Publisher Services